OH SUGAR!

OH SUGAR!

Vie Books is an imprint of Summersdale Publishers Ltd

Summersdale Publishers Ltd
46 West Street
Chichester
West Sussex
PO19 1RP
UK

www.summersdale.com

Printed and bound by CPI Group (UK) Ltd, Croydon, CR0 4YY

ISBN: 978-1-84953-667-7

OH SUGAR!

How to satisfy your sweet tooth naturally for a happy, healthy lifestyle

Katherine Bassford

Disclaimer

Every effort has been made to ensure that the information in this book is accurate and current at the time of publication. The author and the publisher cannot accept responsibility for any misuse or misunderstanding of any information contained herein, or any loss, damage or injury, be it health, financial or otherwise, suffered by any individual or group acting upon or relying on information contained herein. None of the opinions or suggestions in this book are intended to replace medical opinion. If you have concerns about your health, please seek professional advice.

Contents

Introduction..7

My Story..11

Part 1: The Not-So-Sweet Truth.................................15

Chapter 1 – Why is Sugar So Bad For Us?................................16

Chapter 2 – Are You Addicted to Sugar? Take the Test...............28

Part 2: Sugar Facts and Cravings..............................33

Chapter 3 – Sugar FAQs..34

Chapter 4 – Discover How Much Sugar You're Really
Eating (How to Read Food Labels)..43

Chapter 5 – Eight Ways to Satisfy Your Sweet Tooth Naturally....55

Chapter 6 – Three Secret Weapons..67

Part 3: Retrain Your Brain......................................73

Chapter 7 – Be Kind to Yourself and Other Mind-bending Tips.....74

Chapter 8 – Breaking Habits..82

Chapter 9 – Happy Eating..89

Part 4: A Low-Sugar Day..**99**

Chapter 10 – Breakfast..100

Chapter 11 – Mid-morning Munchies.................................115

Chapter 12 – Lunch...125

Chapter 13 – Afternoon Slump...141

Chapter 14 – Dinner...148

Final Thoughts..166

Resources...168

Acknowledgements...170

About the Author..171

Introduction

When a fruit yoghurt contains more sugar than ice cream, and a cereal bar is sweeter than chocolate, you know something's gone badly wrong with our diets. Glance at the ingredients list of the food products you buy and you'll discover sugar is *everywhere*. It lurks in everyday foods such as bread, soup, sauces and salad dressings – and it lurks in gobsmacking amounts. A *Which?* analysis of 100 supermarket cereals found that almost two-thirds contained more sugar per recommended serving than a jam doughnut. (And, let's face it, who sticks to the suggested serving size? Research shows most of us eat at least twice this amount.)

Doughnuts for breakfast does not sound like an auspicious way to start the day! But it gets worse. We know too much sugar makes us fat – that's a given – but it can also make us sick. Increasingly, the signs are that sugar or, more specifically, fructose (one half of table sugar), is the culprit behind rising levels of obesity worldwide and possibly a host of other illnesses too, including heart disease and type 2 diabetes. In the UK we each consume an average of 411 g of added sugar a week – that's almost 100 teaspoons or nearly one small bag of sugar! Over 62 per cent of us are overweight or obese, and it's predicted that five million of us will have diabetes by 2025.

This book aims to put you back in control of your sugar intake, with as little stress as possible. It's purposefully slim on chemistry and big on the thing we're really interested in: the nuts and bolts of how to break a sugar addiction. 'Addiction' may sound a little dramatic, but many of us are dependent on sugar to some degree or other, we just don't know it.

The book is divided into four sections:

Part One explores why sugar is so bad for us and asks 'Are you addicted?' It's the only 'science' chapter in the book, but if you're suffering from information overload you can simply skip to the 'In a nutshell' box at the end of the section and it will tell you all you need to know.

Part Two clears up some pervasive sugar myths and explains how to figure out exactly how much sugar is in the products you buy. This is where you'll also discover eight ways to satisfy your sweet tooth naturally and three simple ways to reduce cravings.

Part Three deals with mindset. We explore a range of ways to recruit your biggest ally (your mind), and we take a step-by-step approach to breaking sugar habits. You'll also discover how a mindful approach can take the stress out of eating (and help you say goodbye to guilt trips).

Part Four outlines a low-sugar day. We'll investigate where sugar lurks in your meals and look at the best low-sugar alternatives (switching to some of these foods can easily halve your sugar intake in a week). At the end of each section, you'll find a handful of delicious low-sugar recipes for inspiration.

Finally, the **Resources** section lists some inspiring books and websites to take a look at if you would like to learn more about some of the topics in this book.

Don't worry, you don't need to do all of this in one go. It's possible to achieve all of the above in small, easy steps…

The small steps approach: why you don't need to cut out all sugar from this moment on

You could wake up tomorrow morning and swear you'll never eat another grain of sugar for the rest of your life. You could also vow that every day you're going to exercise for an hour, meditate for 30 minutes and repeat positive affirmations in the mirror for 15 minutes before going to work… but how long will this regime last?

As a rule, extreme all-or-nothing goals and strict diets are a recipe for failure. When it comes to lasting change, the only thing that works is something you can do each day and continue to do for the rest of your life. That's why this isn't a book about cutting all the sugar out of your diet in one go. If you're the kind of person who isn't fazed by this, then skip to the next chapter! However, if you've tried to stop eating sugar in the past, and failed, you might find the next bit interesting…

I came across the 'small steps' philosophy a few years ago when I read *One Small Step Can Change Your Life* by psychologist Dr Robert Maurer. Dr Maurer is an expert in the psychology of success and lectures on how to make major life changes with minimal disruption. He advises that in order to get yourself to do something you've been avoiding or find overwhelming, you need to make a pact with yourself that you are only going to take a small step. I'm sure you've heard this before, but when I say 'small', I mean the tiniest step known to mankind – one so minuscule it's embarrassing! For example: to create the habit of flossing your teeth, floss one tooth every night; to start exercising regularly, do one press up every day; to stop adding sugar to your cup of tea, remove a few grains from your teaspoon each week. (This is how I went from a 2-teaspoons-of-sugar tea habit down to zero.)

As ridiculous as it sounds, these tiny steps bypass the part of the brain (the amygdala) that triggers the fight-or-flight response whenever it senses danger (real or imagined). This allows you to tiptoe past fear and resistance and take one tentative step after another. You don't need a scientific study to tell you this approach works. Which are you more likely to do: spring clean the whole house, or set a timer for 5 minutes and tidy up one area? Cut out all sugar from this moment on, or buy one less can of fizzy drink a week? The examples might seem silly but the point is, *they get done*. Any behaviour that is repeated frequently lays down new neural pathways in the brain. Day by day, you are building new, healthy eating habits. The process is enjoyable – it doesn't require Herculean effort – ergo, you keep doing it. Before you know it, you're doing the thing you previously thought you couldn't (even if it's something as simple as not adding sugar to your tea). The trick is to choose a first step that is so easy and non-threatening, you cannot fail.

As you read through the rest of the book, make a mental note of some small steps you can take to reduce your sugar intake. If you ever find yourself making excuses, cut back on the size of the step!

My Story

In my teens, before I knew any better, I added 2 teaspoons of sugar to every mug of tea – and it wasn't unheard of for me to drink six mugs of tea a day. That's 12 teaspoons of sugar per day, for years. I shudder when I think about it now, but at the time I thought it was a physical impossibility for me to drink tea that hadn't been sweetened.

A few years later, I started studying experimental psychology at university, learning about the brain and behaviour. Too bad I didn't apply this knowledge to myself! I still added sugar to my tea. I also sprinkled it on my cereal, which I had with a glass of juice every morning. As for my evening meal; let's just say I was no stranger to that classic post-nightclub combination of a pot of instant noodles and a slice of chocolate cake. Strangely, I started to put on weight (2 stone to be precise). If I didn't eat something every few hours, I felt very weird – tired, spaced out, anxious and dizzy.

Fast forward ten years and I am officially into health and fitness. I have weaned myself off sugar in my tea using the small-steps technique and I have switched to a 'healthy' diet. For breakfast I have a bowl of muesli and chopped fruit, with a glass of freshly squeezed juice. When I hit an energy slump a few hours later, I nibble on nuts, dark chocolate and dried fruit. Lunch might be homemade soup and bread, followed by a fruit yoghurt or natural cereal bar. I thought I was eating all the right things. What I didn't realise was that my so-called 'healthy diet' contained a whopping daily dose of up to 30 teaspoons of sugar!

Things change again when a publisher approaches me to write this book. I have now been a health writer and personal trainer for over 12 years. I have said goodbye to refined grains, dried fruit and fruit juice, and I'm eating a diet of meat, fish, eggs, nuts, fruit and lots of vegetables. I feel confident there isn't much room for improvement, but as I learn more about sugar, I tweak my diet:

- I stop eating mountains of fruit every morning and eat more eggs.
- If I have fruit for breakfast, I replace bananas and mangoes with berries and kiwi fruit.
- I stop using balsamic vinegar in my salad dressings every day.
- I stop eating 'natural bars' made from dried fruit.
- I switch to drinking red wine over white.
- I replace the tonic in my gin and tonic with soda water.
- I eat some protein and fat with every meal.
- I start practising mindful eating (see **Chapter 9**).

These are small things. I didn't expect them to make a massive difference, but they honestly did. Within days I felt better; within weeks I couldn't believe the change. My head was clearer, I woke up feeling less groggy, I had more energy, I didn't need snacks between meals, I stopped craving wine in the evenings and I lost over half a stone in weight! In my highly 'scientific' survey of 30 friends, every person who reduced the sugar in their diet, said they experienced the same things too (you'll see their testimonies throughout the book).

I'm not a scientist. And I'm not a nutritionist. I am a consumer who supposedly knew more than the average person (due to my background in health) but it turns out I wasn't doing as well as I thought. Little wonder really; nutrition can be a confusing subject. No one seems to agree on anything! Nutritionists tell you one thing; the government tells you something else. Top experts who have been studying sugar and nutrition for years don't even agree with each other. And let's not get started on food manufacturers' hype about their products. How is the average person supposed to know what to eat?

I hope this book will help you feel more in control. None of this is an exact science; new findings will shed light on sugar and alter current thinking. In the meantime, start taking the simple steps outlined in this book to avoid added sugar and processed food, and you won't go far wrong!

Part 1

THE NOT-SO-SWEET TRUTH

Chapter 1
Why is Sugar So Bad for Us?

It's hard to imagine now, but in the eighteenth century, sugar was a luxury product used only by the wealthy. It was such a prized item that ornate 'sugar boxes', similar to boxes made for jewellery, were created to keep the precious contents under lock and key. Fast-forward 200 years and things couldn't be more different. In the UK, we each consume more than 13 teaspoons of sugar a day on average, with some people consuming up to 46 teaspoons.

Sugar fact

Two centuries ago, we used to eat 1.8–2.2 kg of sugar a year in the UK. That's less than 1½ teaspoons a day. We now consume over 13 teaspoons a day. Americans consume 44 teaspoons a day (68 kg a year), according to the US Department of Agriculture.

The UK is a nation of sweet-lovers:

- In 2013, we each devoured on average 11.2 kg of chocolate (that's the equivalent of eating 266 Mars bars).

- We eat more sweets, cakes and biscuits than any other country in Europe.
- Our soft drink and fruit juice consumption has increased by 30 per cent in the past two decades to 229 litres per person per year. Two-thirds of this is fizzy drinks.

Soft drinks now account for 30 per cent of children's sugar intake. In England, more than a quarter of five year olds suffer from tooth decay and nearly 500 children a week are admitted to hospital with rotten teeth.

It's not just obviously sweet things we need to be wary of though; sugar is hiding in many everyday foods:

Food	Teaspoons of added sugar
Dollop of tomato sauce	1–2
Cereal bar	Up to 8
Serving of muesli	Up to 4
Serving of pasta sauce from a jar	2
Cinnamon latte	6–7
Serving of berry-flavoured water	5
Can of soup	3
Fruit smoothie	6
Probiotic drink	2
Flavoured yoghurt	4–6
Falafel wrap	Up to 2
… the list goes on.	

How much sugar should we be eating?

In 2014, the World Health Organization (WHO) issued new guidelines suggesting that cutting the amount of sugar we eat from the current recommended limit of 10 per cent of our total calorie intake per day to 5 per cent would be beneficial. That's about **25 g or 6 teaspoons*** of sugar per adult per day. This is less than the amount of sugar found in one 50 g chocolate bar or can of fizzy drink.

*The limit includes sugars added to food as well as sugars that are naturally present in honey, syrups, fruit juices and fruit concentrates. It does not include the sugars in fresh fruit, vegetables and milk.

What is sugar?

You would think a definition of sugar would be easy, but just to make things difficult there are several types of sugar, and what scientists call 'sugar' and what we call 'sugar' are two slightly different things:

- What we call sugar (the stuff we put in our food and in our hot drinks), is officially called sucrose.
- When scientists talk about 'blood sugar', they are referring to glucose.

For the average person trying to learn about sugar, this is not spectacularly helpful. (It's also something food manufacturers are all too aware of and will exploit if you're not careful.) Thankfully, you don't need a PhD in biochemistry in order to get to grips with sugar; you just need a few basic facts.

Different sugars

All sugars are carbohydrates. 'Carbohydrate' simply means molecules made from carbon, hydrogen and oxygen.

There are several different types of sugar – glucose, fructose ('fruit sugar'), galactose (forms part of lactose), sucrose ('table sugar'), lactose ('milk sugar') and maltose ('malt sugar').

Don't worry about remembering all the names. For the purpose of this book, the sugars we're really interested in are glucose, fructose and sucrose (table sugar).

- **Glucose** is found naturally in plants (fruit, vegetables, beans and grains).
- **Fructose** is found naturally in fruit and honey, and to a lesser extent, in vegetables.
- **Table sugar (sucrose)** is extracted from sugar cane and sugar beet and contains **50 per cent glucose and 50 per cent fructose**.

Do we need sugar in our diets?

While we need glucose in order for our brain and body to function properly, **we can get all of our daily glucose needs by eating a balanced diet**. Glucose occurs naturally in fruit and vegetables. In addition, a proportion of the protein and fat we consume is changed into glucose once eaten. So, as far as the body is concerned, **all natural food provides glucose**. As author John Yudkin explains, in *Pure, White and Deadly*, 'there is no physiological requirement for sugar… on its own or in any food or drink.' Not only is there no physiological requirement for sugar in our diet, it's actually toxic, especially in the unprecedented amounts we now eat.

Six reasons to avoid sugar

We've grown up being told that sugar is bad for us because it contains 'empty calories' and it's no friend to teeth. But that's just the tip of the iceberg. Evidence is mounting that excessive amounts of sugar wreaks havoc on our metabolism and sets us up for weight gain and many serious diseases. One sugar in particular seems to be especially bad for us. Fructose, found in table sugar and high-fructose corn syrup, behaves in a very different way to any other sugar, as explained below.

This is what excessive sugar in our diet does to us:

1. Sugar makes us eat more

Normally, appetite hormones signal to the brain when we've had enough to eat. But fructose doesn't play by the rules. It doesn't trigger 'stop eating' hormones, so it sneaks in under the radar undetected. This explains why we can munch our way through a whole pack of sweets or biscuits without feeling full.

There's a logical explanation for this: thousands of years ago, our ancestors came across fructose in berries, honey and roots dug up from the ground. As this precious high-energy food was so rare, our bodies evolved with no fructose 'off switch' – so we could eat large amounts. This once nifty survival trait is a big problem now that we're bombarded by fructose in so many foods.

It gets worse: fructose is turned to fat in the body (see point 2) and fat also interferes with our appetite-control system. Hormones that normally tell us when to stop eating, such as cholecystokinin, insulin and leptin, no longer work as well as they should. Result: we feel hungry and end up eating more of **every type of food**, not just sugar!

2. Sugar makes us fat

Fructose is metabolised in a different way to glucose. Whereas glucose is used to fuel every cell in the body, most of the fructose we eat shoots straight to the liver where it is converted to fat (triglycerides). This fat either stays in the liver, where it can build up and cause non-alcoholic fatty liver disease (NAFLD), or it gets released into the bloodstream, increasing our risk of obesity, heart disease and stroke. Fructose metabolism also creates a long list of waste products and toxins, including uric acid. Uric acid can crystallise and cause gout. It also makes blood vessels less elastic, raising blood pressure, and increasing the risk of heart disease and stroke.

The worldwide obesity problem has been accelerating in direct proportion to consumption of sugar. In the UK, one in three children leaving primary school are overweight or obese. In America, the situation is even worse. It's thought that up to 24 per cent of the children there have NAFLD.

'Fat' thin people

Just because you don't look overweight, doesn't mean you're out of the woods. Many people look healthy and trim on the outside but are carrying excess fat on the inside. Excess sugar tends to be stored as fat in the abdominal region and around organs such as the heart, liver, kidneys and pancreas. This abdominal or 'visceral fat' is the worst kind of fat, because it produces inflammatory molecules that enter your bloodstream and can trigger a wide range of diseases including heart disease, hypertension and type 2 diabetes. It's thought up to 50 per cent of 'normal weight' women and 20 per cent of men are actually obese based on their visceral fat. Do you have visceral fat? One of the indications doctors look out for is a pot belly or 'muffin top'!

3. Sugar causes insulin resistance

During digestion, food and drink are broken down into glucose. In response to rising blood sugar levels, the pancreas secretes a hormone called insulin. Insulin acts like a key that unlocks the door into cells such as muscle cells, so that glucose can be taken on as fuel. If we keep eating sugary food, the body tries desperately to keep up by producing more and more insulin. Eventually, the pancreas gets worn out and stops producing insulin, or our cells become numb to insulin and we become insulin resistant. Result: raised, and potentially toxic blood sugar levels.

While further research is required before we can say that excess sugar actually causes type 2 diabetes, there is a high correlation between countries with the highest sugar consumption and deaths from diabetes. Less than 30 years ago, type 2 diabetes was virtually unheard of. Now it affects 300 million people worldwide. In the UK, seven million people are estimated to have prediabetes (this is the 'grey area' between normal blood sugar and diabetic blood sugar levels).

Remember I said fructose behaves differently to other sugars? As fructose is metabolised by the liver, it does not directly cause blood sugar levels to rise. However, it increases circulating fatty acids and this excess fat interferes with insulin's 'lock' mechanism. This means insulin struggles to remove glucose from the bloodstream. End result: increased blood sugar levels.

How junk food makes you want to eat more

Endocrinologist and obesity expert Robert H. Lustig says it's insulin that drives weight gain. Here's how: leptin is a hormone which goes from our fat cells to our brain and tells it that we have enough energy stored and we can stop eating. More fat equals more leptin. As the fat cells of overweight and obese people get bigger, they produce higher levels of leptin, which should, logically, regulate appetite; so what's going wrong? The answer is that the body has developed leptin resistance, and Dr Lustig explains that insulin is to blame.

As explained above, a high-sugar, processed and junk-food diet stimulates raised blood sugar levels and therefore, lots of insulin. Insulin's job is to tell the body to store this energy, either as muscle glycogen or fat. But this is the real kicker: excess insulin blocks leptin in the brain – so the brain doesn't receive the message that the body's fat cells have enough energy stored and we can stop eating. In short, says Dr Lustig, 'the higher your insulin goes, the more energy you store [fat] and the hungrier you get.'

4. Sugar raises your risk of chronic disease

Excess sugar consumption is now thought to underlie many diseases prevalent in Europe and North America. Two of the leading causes of death in the UK are heart disease and cancer:

- A major US study by the Harvard School of Public Health found that people who received more than a quarter of their daily calories through added sugar were almost three times more likely to die of cardiovascular disease than those consuming less than a quarter of their calories from sugar.

- In a study published in the *American Journal of Clinical Nutrition*, drinking two or more fizzy or syrup-based drinks each day was linked to a 90 per cent extra risk of developing pancreatic cancer.

- Cancerous cells consume much more glucose than normal cells. We don't know whether a high-sugar diet causes cancer, just that cancer cells consume much more glucose than normal cells in order to sustain their growth. A recent UCLA study also showed that cancerous pancreatic cells use fructose to feed tumour growth.

- More than a quarter of all deaths in the UK are caused by heart and circulatory diseases, and every 2 minutes someone in the UK is diagnosed with cancer.

Sugar fact

PET scans (positron emission tomography) are used to detect the presence and severity of cancers. They work on the basis that cancer cells consume glucose at a much faster rate than normal cells. Patients are given an intravenous injection of radioactive glucose, and the scan then detects glucose 'hot spots'. The areas where glucose is being metabolised the fastest in their body are most likely to be cancerous.

5. Sugar affects the brain

Most of us are aware that having a sweet tooth can be disastrous for our waistlines and health. But did you know that sugar can also affect your emotions and mental health? The brain depends on an even supply of glucose to function.

Excess sugar consumption has been implicated in a wide range of psychological problems, including:

- Anxiety
- Depression
- Aggression
- Hyperactivity
- Impaired thinking
- Diminished attention span
- Problems concentrating
- Impaired memory and learning

Research into how sugar affects the brain is still in its early stages, but it's thought that sugar damages the brain's blood vessels and can cause brain shrinkage. In a study of 2,000 people over five years, those with higher glucose levels were 18 per cent more likely to develop dementia (further research needs to be done before we can conclusively say sugar causes these diseases, but there appears to be a strong link*). In August 2009, UCLA researchers discovered that the brains of overweight and obese people look between eight and 16 years older than the brains of those the same age and of healthy weight, and also have less brain tissue. There may even be a relationship between the size of your belly and the structure of your brain! It seems the larger a person's waist-to-hip ratio, the smaller the hippocampus, the brain's memory centre. As your hippocampus shrinks, your memory does too.

*'Glucose Levels and Risk of Dementia', *The New England Journal of Medicine* (2013).

Is sugar making you anxious?

Sugar doesn't necessarily cause anxiety, but it can worsen anxiety symptoms and impair your ability to cope with stress. For example, a sugar high and subsequent crash can cause shaking, difficulty thinking and fatigue – which can contribute to feelings of panic and tension and make anxiety worse.

6. Sugar is addictive

Eat a spoonful of chocolate cake and your brain will do a little happy dance. Sugar stimulates taste receptors on your tongue, which send a signal to the cerebral cortex in the brain. This triggers the release of dopamine, which makes us feel good – cue more chocolate cake. As variety in our diet means we're more likely to get all the nutrients we need, the brain has evolved to pay special attention to new or different tastes. This means that if we eat sugary food day after day, less and less dopamine is released and we need more and more sugary food to get the same warm, fuzzy feeling. This is how sugar becomes addictive (some scientists say it's as addictive as cocaine). The more sugar you eat, the more you crave. If you have a healthy, low-sugar diet and eat the odd piece of chocolate cake once in a blue moon, it won't have the same effect. (Broccoli doesn't trigger a cascade of dopamine – what a surprise.)

'My worst sugar habits are when eating a biscuit with my tea, I cannot stop at one – I have to eat two or more.'
Zeba

'I find that once I open a bag of sweets, they are completely addictive and it's very difficult to stop!'
Eileen

In a nutshell: why is sugar so bad for us?

Scientists are still investigating how sugar affects the body and mind but think a number of factors are at work:

1. Fructose, a main ingredient of table sugar, bypasses the hormonal 'off switch' which tells us when we've had enough to eat
2. Fructose gets sent straight to the liver where it gets turned into fat
3. Sugar can cause insulin resistance, which means insulin can't do its job of removing glucose from the bloodstream, resulting in high blood sugar
4. High blood sugar increases your risk of many chronic diseases
5. Sugar affects the brain and can increase anxiety, depression and hyperactivity
6. Sugar can be highly addictive

Note: This is essentially a dosage issue. Small doses of sugar, such as the natural sugar found in fruits, won't cause the health issues mentioned in this list. Large doses over time (as found in a typical Western diet) can be highly toxic.

Chapter 2
Are You Addicted to Sugar? Take the Test

It's obvious we're eating sugar when we add a teaspoonful to a cup of tea, but with so much sugar hidden in many of our daily foods, it's easy to become hooked without realising it. Feeling sleepy during the day? Mind feeling foggy? These could be signs that your body is not tolerating the amount of sugar in your system.

To find out if you could be addicted to sugar, answer the questions below:

1. Do you find it difficult to walk past a sugary treat, such as a plate of biscuits, without taking one?
2. After eating a piece of chocolate or a biscuit, do you find it hard to resist eating more?
3. After meals do you crave something sweet?
4. Do your energy levels rise after eating, but crash an hour or two later?
5. Do you regularly feel drowsy during the day?
6. Does your mind often feel foggy and not very sharp?

7. Are you a bit plump around the middle?
8. If you try to give up sugar, or are forced to go without it for a day, do you feel irritable and anxious?
9. Do you feel panicky if you don't have any 'treats' in the house?
10. Do you think about sugary foods several times a day and plan when you're going to eat them?

These are all signs that your body is struggling to keep your blood sugar levels stable. If you answered 'yes' to several (or all) of the questions, you're likely to be experiencing strong sugar cravings and could be addicted. That's the bad news. The good news is that when you reduce your sugar intake, there's a long list of life-enhancing benefits you can look forward to.

The benefits of going sugar free:

- More energy
- Fewer (or no) cravings
- A clearer mind
- A more balanced mood
- Weight loss
- Younger looking skin
- More restful sleep
- Reduced risk of tooth decay
- Reduced risk of developing health problems, including many chronic diseases

'When I cut the sugar out, I felt amazing and my energy levels were sky high.'
Mike

'My skin definitely improved. I know my mood improved too.'
Georgina

'I feel wonderful. I sleep well and I'm not as dehydrated and groggy as I sometimes used to feel.'
Joanne

'I instantly lost weight and now have more motivation to do sporty things.'
Jason

'I feel less tired, I don't crave alcohol and I weigh the same as I did 45 years ago!'
Roger

'I've stopped having cravings and hunger pangs during the day.'
Jo

'I've definitely got more energy, more thinking time and I feel less sluggish. Weight loss goes hand in hand with this, absolutely.'
Tom

Keeping a food diary

If the questions above were tricky to answer, you might find it useful to keep a food and mood diary for a week. This can reveal surprising patterns and connections between what you eat and how you feel. Do negative feelings and emotions increase after eating sugary food, for example?

There are several chapters coming up which will help you identify where sugar hides in your diet (see **Chapter 3** – Sugar FAQs and **chapters 10–14** which look at different mealtimes and snacks), but for now the following list will give you a good idea of what could be affecting your mood. Keep this list in mind when making your diary notes.

Main sources of fructose in our diet

Sugary drinks (e.g. soft drinks, fizzy drinks, fruit juice, energy drinks, alcohol)

Added sugar (e.g. table sugar, honey, maple syrup)

High-fructose corn syrup (in processed foods)

Refined carbohydrates (e.g. bread, cereals, crisps, pastries, cakes, biscuits, pies)

Ready-made meals and takeaways

Fruit

Sugar from grains and refined carbohydrates

While this book focuses on reducing table sugar and fructose in your diet, for optimal health, you may also want to consider reducing the amount of grains you eat, particularly if you eat grains several times a day. Carbohydrates that have been refined – such as crisps, crackers, bread, pasta, rice and cereal – have had much of their fibre stripped away (along with many nutrients). This means they are digested quickly and are rapidly converted to glucose. Unless you are very active, and use up the excess glucose, these foods can raise blood sugar and insulin levels, promoting fat storage and other health problems associated with high blood sugar. Wholegrain versions tend to contain more nutrients as well as fibre, which helps you to feel full, so these are better options to go for. However, many have a similar impact on blood glucose levels as the refined 'white' versions. For example, wholewheat bread spikes blood sugar just as quickly as white bread.

Part 2

SUGAR FACTS AND CRAVINGS

Chapter 3
Sugar FAQs

The topic of eating less sugar naturally triggers lots of questions. How far across the board do you need to go with this? There's a bewildering array of sweeteners to choose from. Should you switch to brown sugar? Is honey a better alternative? What about agave or artificial sweeteners? This chapter should help clear up any confusion.

Sugar is natural, isn't it?

Table sugar is 'natural' in the sense that it comes from a plant (sugar cane or sugar beet), but 'natural' implies we are eating it in its innate state, which couldn't be further from the truth. The refined white granules we add to our food are a far cry from the natural sugar in a sugar cane stem. Numerous chemicals used in the refining process strip raw sugar of its natural vitamins and minerals (see diagram). Regardless of whether sugar is natural or not, there's one argument no one can quibble with: the amount of sugar in our diets is decidedly *unnatural*.

A quick lesson in how to make table sugar from sugar cane:

First, extract the juice from sugar cane stems by rolling them between heavy rollers.

The juice will contain soil and plant fibre, so add some calcium hydroxide to clean it and then boil it to kill off any enzymes.

Place the syrup in a series of evaporators to remove the water and concentrate the sugar crystals.

Congratulations – you now have 'raw sugar'!

But there's one problem; your sugar crystals are brown. Immerse your sugar crystals in a concentrated syrup to soften them, then dissolve in water and pass through charcoal; this will remove their coloured outer coating.

Boil again until the sugar crystallises, and place in a giant centrifuge. The syrup (blackstrap molasses) will be forced out through the perforations and…

… *voilà*, perfect white sugar!

Is brown sugar better than white sugar?

It's tempting to think that brown sugar is healthier than white sugar, but sadly this isn't the case. Brown sugar is either unrefined sugar which has some residual molasses in it, or it's a fake (i.e. it's really refined sugar which has had molasses added back in to give it an appealing colour and flavour). 'Dark brown sugar' contains more molasses than 'light brown sugar', hence the difference in colour.

What about 'raw', 'unrefined', or 'natural' brown sugar?

'Raw' sugars such as 'light muscovado', 'muscovado' and 'Demerara' are not raw at all. They are partially refined. During the manufacturing process, sugar is repeatedly boiled and crystallised. Each successive crystallisation has a higher concentration of molasses trapped in the sugar crystals. The first crystallisation produces a light coloured sugar (Demerara), the second crop of crystals is slightly darker (light muscovado), and the third crop is darker still (muscovado). Molasses does contain nutrients, but the amount we're talking about is negligible. In summary, your body doesn't care; it's still sugar and it will still have the same destructive effects!

Surely honey is all right? It's from nature!

This is where things get tricky. Honey tends to have slightly less of an effect on blood glucose levels than sugar. It also contains antioxidants, enzymes, vitamins and minerals, and has antibacterial and anti-inflammatory properties. The problem is, honey is 80 per cent sugar (fructose and glucose). Worse, its fructose content is 40 per cent. So in terms of fructose intake, there's really not much difference between eating a spoonful of table sugar and a spoonful of honey.

True, our ancestors ate honey. But they ate it very rarely and had to work hard to get it (walking for miles and shinnying up trees to get to bees' nests). The raw honey they ate was also vastly different to the honey we eat today. The jars of honey we buy from supermarkets are heavily processed and subject to excessive heating – to the point where honey's nutritional and medicinal properties are drastically reduced, or have given up the ghost altogether.

So, should you eat honey? Some experts stipulate total abstinence, while others take a more laid-back approach. I think the answer is 'it depends':

- If you are healthy, don't need to lose weight *and* you have a fairly low sugar diet, then the odd bit of honey shouldn't be a problem. Just use it sparingly.
- If you are overweight or have blood sugar issues, it may be advisable to keep your honey intake to an absolute minimum.
- If you decide to eat honey, go for the high-quality stuff. Buy raw honey (unfiltered and unheated) or unprocessed manuka honey. This way, at least you're consuming some nutrients alongside the sugar.
- What the bees feed on determines the level of antioxidants in the honey. Generally speaking, darker honeys, such as buckwheat honey, contain more antioxidants.

Can I eat agave nectar instead?

Agave syrup is advertised as being 'natural' but the reality is, it is highly processed, it has no health benefits and it is up to 90 per cent fructose – *worse than table sugar and high-fructose corn syrup.*

You'll often see agave being touted as being a 'low-GI' sugar. The reason agave ranks low on the glycaemic index is because it contains so much fructose. Fructose, as we know, is not metabolised well by the body and goes straight to the liver, so it doesn't cause raised blood glucose. For this reason, be extra wary of 'low-GI' jams and spreads – the easiest way to make something low GI is to pack it full of fructose, often disguised as 'grape concentrate'.

Coconut sugar?

Avoid high-sugar sweeteners such as **golden syrup**, commercial **maple syrup**, **coconut sugar** (coconut palm sugar), **coconut syrup** and **coconut nectar**. All are around 40 per cent fructose.

The reason raw coconut is fine to eat (i.e. flakes, flour, desiccated) is because it's the flesh of the coconut. Coconut sugar, syrup and nectar on the other hand are made from the sap of the coconut tree, which is boiled to create a syrup that is 70–80 per cent sucrose – half of which is fructose!

Dried fruit and sun-dried tomatoes?

The reason dried fruit tastes so good is because it's 50–70 per cent sugar, a large proportion of which is fructose. Raisins, for example, are 38 per cent fructose and 20 per cent glucose. Similarly, drying a tomato concentrates its natural sugars; a raw tomato is 2.6 per cent sugar, whereas a sun-dried tomato is 38 per cent sugar.

These percentages can seem a bit confusing at first. Surely a tomato contains the same amount of sugar whether it's fresh or dried? When the water content of fruit is removed, fruit shrinks by about three-quarters. Dried fruit contains the same amount of sugar per fruit as the fresh version... the issue here is **portion control**. Dried fruit is less filling than fresh fruit due to its lack of water. Most of us would baulk at eating ten fresh apricots in one sitting, but we wouldn't think twice about eating ten dried apricots.

Check out the sugar content of dried fruit below (as you do, bear in mind that a standard chocolate bar is around 60 per cent sugar).

Dried fruit	Sugar content (approx.)
Sultana	73 per cent
Cranberry*	65 per cent
Date	65 per cent
Currant	63 per cent
Apple	62 per cent
Fig	53 per cent
Apricot	40 per cent
Prune (dried plum)	31 per cent

Source: NUTTAB Food Standards Australia New Zealand

*Many dried fruits have sugar added to them. Dried cranberries would taste very tart if they weren't sweetened.

Bearing in mind the above, either omit dried fruit from your diet altogether (especially if you consume a lot of fructose from other sources, such as fruit juice), or treat it as an occasional indulgence rather than something to be consumed every day. Whatever you do, keep an eye on your portions!

Sugar fact

If you snack on a handful of dates (45 g) you might just as well have eaten a chocolate bar in terms of your sugar intake (around 7 teaspoons)!

What's high-fructose corn syrup (HFCS)?

High-fructose corn syrup (also known as **'glucose-fructose syrup'** in the UK) is a highly sweet, gloopy syrup which is manufactured from corn syrup by converting a large proportion of its glucose into fructose. Manufacturers around the world are switching to it in droves because it's cheaper than sugar and it extends the shelf life of products. As a result, we are consuming HFCS in ever-increasing quantities and scientists are concerned about the impact on our health.

As the name suggests, high-fructose corn syrup contains high levels of fructose. It is 55 per cent fructose and 42 per cent glucose (i.e. slightly higher in fructose than table sugar and with roughly the same fructose content as honey). The manufacture of HFCS also involves the use of artificial and synthetic agents, which may be harmful to health. HFCS in diets has been linked to cardiovascular disease, diabetes and non-alcoholic fatty liver disease. It is thought to be highly addictive and it is currently being blamed for the obesity epidemic in America, where it can be found in every processed food and sugar-sweetened drink. (Note: HFCS is not the same as 'corn syrup', a syrup made from corn starch, which is 100 per cent glucose.)

Where to spot it: You'll commonly find HFCS in cereal bars, doughnuts, chocolate bars, biscuits and ice cream.

Can I switch to artificial sweeteners instead?

Artificial sweeteners are several times sweeter than table sugar, so less is required to sweeten food, which sounds promising. However, they are relative newcomers to our diet, so it's hard to know whether they're safe for long-term human consumption. Scientific evidence for the health benefits of artificial sweeteners has shown mixed findings. We simply don't know how large doses of these chemicals will affect the body over the course of a lifetime. Aspartame, the most extensively studied artificial sweetener, has been linked to headaches, dizziness, weight gain, depression and brain cancer. The European Food Safety Authority (EFSA) assessed the evidence and concluded that aspartame is safe and poses no threat to health 'at current levels of exposure'. However, many scientists are still concerned and say artificial sweeteners:

May lead to weight gain

Obesity levels have rocketed since diet drinks and snacks have been available and some large studies show that switching to these sweeteners does not lead to weight loss – in humans or animals. The cause isn't known but may be linked to the two theories below.

May increase your cravings for sugar

Artificial sweeteners are several hundred times sweeter than sucrose, but don't contain any calories. It's possible that a sweet taste without the calories doesn't satisfy our innate desire for sweetness, so we keep craving more.

May adversely affect blood sugar and insulin levels

We don't really know how the body responds to being primed for an influx of sugar and calories that never arrive. One theory is that the sweet taste of artificial sweeteners alerts the brain to get ready for incoming sugar. In preparation for the expected surge, *real* sugar is absorbed from the bloodstream, triggering insulin production and turning sugar into fat.

The four main artificial sweeteners are **saccharin**, **cyclamate**, **aspartame** (marketed as NutraSweet) and **sucralose**. You will frequently see them cropping up in carbonated soft drinks, especially 'diet' versions.

Some manufacturers have switched to using sugar alcohols (a type of alcohol prepared from sugar) such as **sorbitol**, **maltitol**, **mannitol**, **xylitol**. Sugar alcohols do not cause tooth cavities so are often used in sugar-free gum. However, as with artificial sweeteners they affect blood sugar levels indirectly and also have an unfortunate side effect. Sugar alcohols are not absorbed by the gut and in large doses, can cause bloating and diarrhoea. Of all the sugar alcohols, the body seems to tolerate xylitol in small amounts.

If you are keen to use sweeteners, I recommend sticking to the advice offered by the Harvard School of Public Health: 'For adults trying to wean themselves from sugary soda, diet soda is a possible short-term substitute, best used in small amounts over a short period of time. For children, the long-term effects of consuming artificially sweetened beverages are unknown, so it's best for kids to avoid them.'

This is beginning to get on my nerves – is there anything sweet I *can* eat?!

Yes! There are healthier, natural alternatives to sugar – see **Chapter 5** – Eight Ways to Satisfy Your Sweet Tooth Naturally.

Chapter 4

Discover How Much Sugar You're Really Eating (How to Read Food Labels)

> *'I have found it a real struggle to give up sugar;*
> *mainly because it is in EVERYTHING!'*
> Rachael

With sugar present in so many supermarket products, there's a simple way to reduce the amount of sugar in your diet: avoid all processed food! Simple, but not necessarily easy. At the very least, sniff out the worst offenders and boot them from your trolley. It takes seconds to read a food label once you get used to it and it will give you a feeling of power (sort of).

Reading food labels

If you pick up a tin or carton of food and glance at the sugars listed on the food label, you'll see there's a slight hitch in our plan. Food manufacturers are not legally required to specify the type of sugar in their product. As a result, all we get to go by is a figure under the heading 'Carbohydrate (of which sugars)'. This means that when a label says 'sugars' it's potentially referring to all types of sugar – naturally occurring (from fruit and milk) and added. Handy, huh? That's why it's a good idea to resort to Plan B and check the ingredients list for anything nasty lurking there (more on this in a moment).

Nutrition information			
Typical values	Per 100 g	Per 1/4 pot	% based on GDA for women
Energy	256 kj 61 kcal	320 kj 76 kcal	3.8 %
Protein	4.9 g	6.1 g	13.6 %
Carbohydrate of which **sugars** of which starch	6.9 g 6.9 g nil	8.6 g 8.6 g nil	3.7 % 9.6 % -
Fat of which **saturates** mono-unsaturates polyunsaturates	1.5 g 0.9 g 0.4 g nil	1.9 g 1.1 g 0.5 g nil	2.7 % 5.5 % - -
Fibre	nil	nil	nil
Salt of which sodium	0.2 g trace	0.3 g 0.1 g	5.0 % 4.2 %
Vitamins & minerals	% of RDA Recommended daily amount		
Calcium	168 mg	210 mg	26 %

If a food product contains less than 5 g of sugar per 100 g it is considered to be low in sugar. If a product contains more than 15 g of sugar per 100 g it is considered to be high in sugar.

How to calculate how many teaspoons of sugar there are in a serving

The percentage rule is handy for making quick decisions as to whether to buy or avoid a certain product but, personally, I prefer to visualise how many teaspoons of sugar there are in a serving. It somehow makes the sugar content more real. It's easy to work out:

- The first thing you need to know is that a teaspoon of sugar weighs 4.2 g.
- Next, check the food label to see how many grams of sugar are under the 'per serving' column (in the previous example, it's 'per ¼ pot').
- Divide this figure by 4.2 to get the number of teaspoons of sugar in a serving (if you don't have a calculator to hand, roughly divide the figure by four).
- The product in the previous example contains just over 2 teaspoons of sugar (8.6 divided by 4.2).

Bear in mind that a manufacturer's idea of what constitutes a 'serving' or a 'portion' can often be wildly different to yours, so adjust accordingly. Labels on cans or bottles of drink often list the sugar content under 'per 100 ml'. However, a standard can of drink is around 330 ml, which means you need to multiply the sugar 'per 100 ml' figure by 3.3. If you don't do this you'll be seriously underestimating how much sugar you're consuming!

Remember; new World Health Organization guidelines recommend adults consume no more than 6 teaspoons of sugar a day.

The one exception: dairy

Just when you think you've got your head around all this, there's an anomaly you need to be aware of. If you look at the food label for whole milk (cow, goat or sheep) you'll see that it contains 4.7 g of sugar per 100 ml. If you're a big milk drinker, you might work this out and get a fright: a litre of milk contains just over 11 teaspoons of sugar! However, the sugar in milk is a naturally occurring sugar called lactose. In the body, lactose is broken down into glucose and galactose. Milk is therefore fructose-free.

This means that when you're working out how much sugar is in a milk drink, you can **ignore the first 4.7 g of sugar** per 100 ml. You can safely assume that any figure over 4.7 g is **added sugar**. For example, if your child's favourite chocolate milk drink contains 13 g of sugar per 100 ml, you know there is 8.3 g of added sugar per 100 ml (13 g–4.7 g of lactose = 8.3 g). To convert this into teaspoons, divide 8.3 g by 4.2 and you know the drink contains 1.9 teaspoons of added sugar.

Other dairy products, such as cheese, cream, butter and yoghurt, contain varying amounts of lactose, depending on processing methods. Hard cheeses and butter contain the least lactose.

Food label summary

RULE 1: Eat products with less than 5 g of sugar per 100 g

Stick to products that are less than 5 per cent sugar (i.e. less than 5 g per 100 g). If a product contains over 15 g of sugar per 100 g, it's a high-sugar food.

Remember: the maximum recommended daily intake of sugar per adult per day is 6 teaspoons.

RULE 2: Drink products with 0 g sugar per 100 ml

That's not a typo! When sugar is in liquid form, its negative effects are magnified. The lack of fibre in the liquid means the sugar gets absorbed and sent to the liver very quickly, leading to fat storage and liver overload (see box at end of chapter for more information). The number one thirst-quencher to turn to is water. If you're not keen on plain water, drink sparkling water or herbal tea. Tea and coffee can count towards your water intake, but as caffeine can stimulate an insulin response, limit caffeinated drinks such as tea, coffee and green tea to two cups a day. If you drink juice, drink it very occasionally.

Reading the ingredients list

A quick way to check a product for added sugar is to read the ingredients list. Manufacturers don't like to make this too easy for us – they sneak sugar into their products in various guises. Did you know there are now 40 different types of sugar used in processed food? Unless you're blessed with a photographic memory (I'm not), keeping track of these various sugars can be a challenge. Here are some of the different types of sugar to look out for:

- Agave syrup or nectar*
- Barley malt
- Beet sugar*
- Blackstrap molasses*
- Brown sugar*
- Cane crystals*
- Cane sugar*
- Cane juice*
- Caramel*
- Caster sugar*

- Coconut sugar or coconut palm sugar*
- Corn syrup
- Demerara sugar*
- Dextrin
- Dextrose (another name for glucose)
- Fruit juice concentrate (often grape as it's so sweet)*
- Fructose* (fruit sugar)
- Galactose
- Glucose (another name for dextrose)
- Golden syrup*
- High-fructose corn syrup*
- Honey*
- Icing sugar*
- Invert sugar*
- Lactose (milk sugar)
- Malt syrup
- Maltose (malt sugar)
- Maltodextrin
- Maple syrup*
- Molasses*
- Muscovado sugar*
- Raw sugar*
- Rice syrup (or brown rice syrup)
- Saccharose (another name for sucrose)*
- Sucrose (table sugar)*
- Syrup*
- Treacle*
- Turbinado sugar*

* Contains fructose

Common sugar substitutes:

- Aspartame
- Cyclamate
- Saccharin
- Sucralose

- Stevia
- Sugar alcohols: xylitol, maltitol, mannitol and sorbitol

Watch out for the following warning signs:

- **Sugar listed as the first or second ingredient**
  In an ingredients list, ingredients must be listed in order of weight, with the main ingredient first. If sugar appears as the first or second ingredient, steer clear.

- **Lots of different sugars**
  Food manufacturers know we check to see if sugar is listed high up in the ingredients list and sneakily avoid having to put sugar as the top ingredient by using multiple forms of sugar and listing each one individually. As the sugar content is spread across several different types of sugar, they are used in smaller amounts and can legitimately be listed lower down the ingredients list.

- **'Syrup', 'sweetener', or any word ending in '-ose'**
  As a general rule, if you see the words 'syrup', 'sweetener' or anything ending in '-ose', you can assume it's sugar.

Sugar content in fruit

You don't need to walk round with a calculator working out how much sugar is in every piece of fruit, but it is useful to get an overall picture of which fruits are high in fructose. It's no surprise that many of our favourite fruits happen to be the sweetest:

Low-fructose fruit	High-fructose fruit
Apricot	Grape
Kiwi	Apple
Raspberry	Pear
Strawberry	Mango
Grapefruit	Cherry
Honeydew melon	Banana
Lemon	Lychee
Lime	

However, choosing which fruits to eat is not just a matter of selecting those with the lowest fructose content, there are other factors to consider:

- **The sweeter a fruit tastes, the more fructose it is likely to contain.**

- **The riper the fruit, the more fructose it is likely to contain.** As fruit ripens it converts glucose to fructose, which is why ripe bananas taste sweeter than unripe ones.

- **Different species of the same fruit contain varying amounts of fructose.** For example, an average Golden Delicious apple contains more fructose than a Granny Smith.

- **Fibre content varies a lot between fruits.** Fibre-rich fruit breaks down more slowly in the body. A pear contains more fructose than an orange, but it contains more fibre, so overall, it's the better choice.

- **Some fruits contain more vitamins and antioxidants than others.** The health benefits of many fruits outweigh their high fructose content. Apples, for example, are rich in beneficial phytonutrients, antioxidants, fibre and water. Eating apples has been linked to lowering the risk of chronic diseases including type 2 diabetes, cancer, heart disease and dementia.

This brings us back to the same question: what's the best fruit to eat? As you might have gathered, there is no conclusive answer. The one thing that most people seem to agree on is that when you weigh up both nutrition and fructose content, berries come out on top.

So here's my take on fruit: don't get too hung up on it! Fruit has been in our diets since we were primates. We are designed to process the fructose in fruit, **just not in excessive amounts** (i.e. not in conjunction with our modern day high-sugar, refined diets). If you have no blood sugar issues and are able to eat fructose without any digestive problems, then around two pieces of fruit a day is fine. Fruit should be a supplement rather than the main part of your diet. In other words, avoid eating it for breakfast AND drinking juice AND snacking on dried fruit and fresh fruit throughout the day.

What is a 'serving' or 'portion' of fruit?

It can be bewildering being told to eat 'two pieces of fruit a day' without any further guidance; where does this leave small fruit like cherries or large fruit such as melons? Good question. One serving of fruit for an adult is around 80 g. There's an easy way to remember this:

One serving of fruit for an adult = one piece of fruit about the size of a tennis ball
OR Two pieces of fruit, each about the size of an egg
OR A handful of grapes.

If you'd like to be more specific, you can use the table below as a guide:

Fresh fruit	One serving or portion
Large fruit: Apple, orange, banana, pear, nectarine, peach	1 medium fruit
Medium fruit: Satsuma, tangerine, clementine, kiwi, plum, fig	2 small fruit
Small fruit: Apricot, date, prune Cherries	3 fruit 14 fruit
Pineapple	1 large slice
Melon	1 slice (2 inches)
Papaya and mango	2 slices (2 inches)
Berries and grapes	1 handful (e.g. 10 blackberries)
Grapefruit	½ a medium fruit
Avocado	½ a medium fruit
Tomato	1 medium or 7 cherries
Puréed apple	2 heaped tablespoons

Source: NHS & Dr Mercola

Fruit summary

RULE 1: Aim for two pieces of fruit a day (your body should be able to tolerate more if you are active and have a very low-sugar, unprocessed diet).

RULE 2: If you have health issues*, are overweight, and/or eat a diet high in other sources of fructose such as high-fructose corn syrup in processed food, it could be beneficial to reduce your fruit consumption to one piece of fruit a day, or less.

*E.g. blood sugar problems and fructose intolerance (difficulty digesting fructose).

Note: The NHS advises that children should eat at least five portions of a variety of fruit and vegetables a day. As a rough guide, one portion is the amount they can fit in the palm of their hand.

Why is whole fruit better than fruit juice (and fizzy drinks)?

There's no doubt about it, fruit contains sugar. An apple contains around 3 teaspoons of sugar (just over half of which is fructose) and a banana contains around 4–5 teaspoons. However, nature has created a perfect package. Whole fruits are loaded with fibre, which slows down the rate at which sugar enters the bloodstream. They also contain potent compounds, which have been shown to improve our health and protect against disease. The fructose in fruit bypasses our appetite-control mechanisms, but the fibre makes us feel full and can help insulin do its work. All in all, it's a perfectly balanced system. The liver can easily metabolise small amounts of fructose (i.e. two pieces of fruit) without being overloaded. The proviso to this is: don't *drink* your fruit.

Drinking a glass of fruit juice is the equivalent of consuming several pieces of fruit in a short space of time, without the fibre. A glass of apple juice (freshly squeezed or otherwise) contains around 8 teaspoons of sugar, the same as a glass of Coke. It also contains the same number of calories.

However, it's not just the *amount* of sugar that's a concern. As fruit juice and soft drinks (squashes and fizzy drinks) are sugar in liquid form, large amounts of sugar hit the liver at speed and are converted into fatty acids, which can increase your risk of developing diabetes, cardiovascular disease and liver disease. To make matters worse, as there's no fibre or chewing to slow down consumption, it's easy to consume large portions of fruit juice and soft drinks very quickly. Plus you're bathing your teeth in sugar solution. Bacteria in our mouths feed off sugar and produce an acid. The longer the acid is in contact with the teeth, the worse the risk of tooth decay. The sugars in whole fruit are less likely to cause tooth decay because the sugar is contained within the structure of the fruit.

> In a nutshell, eat your fruit whole and steer clear of fruit juice and soft or fizzy drinks. Studies show one sugary drink a day can raise your risk of diabetes and heart disease by 20 per cent.

Chapter 5
Eight Ways to Satisfy Your Sweet Tooth Naturally

As you eat less sugar and your blood sugar levels become more stable, your cravings and urges to snack should start to disappear (along with other unsavoury symptoms such as tiredness and mood swings). Your taste buds might undergo a similar transformation – foods you previously thought were bland, may start to taste sweet and satisfying, and sugary food and drink, which before were not an issue, may begin to taste super-sweet.

> 'One of the benefits of reducing my sugar intake has been an increased sensitivity to natural sugars. Fruit is really sweet.'
> Katie

> 'When I was diagnosed with type 2 diabetes, I cut down on sugary things. I found it difficult to drink coffee without sugar but I would never spoil my coffee with sugar now!'
> Roger

The following eight foods are naturally sweet and healthy to boot:

1. Coconut

There's a reason tropical islanders call coconut the 'tree of life'. For centuries they have been relying on it as a source of food and medicine, but we're only just cottoning on to its benefits. Coconut is a highly nutritious source of energy; packed with fibre, vitamins and minerals. But the bit that interests researchers the most is its saturated fat content (it's OK; it's the good stuff). The bulk of this fat is lauric acid, a medium-chain fatty acid (MCFA) with special properties. As these fatty acid molecules are quite small, they are easily digested and are sent directly to the liver where they are converted into energy rather than being stored as fat. As this process doesn't require insulin, eating coconut won't cause an insulin spike. To top it all off, coconut is virtually fructose-free. What's not to like?

Eat the raw flesh from a coconut or buy it in the form of flakes, flour, oil, milk, cream or butter:

Coconut flakes: Great for snacking on or sprinkling over desserts.

Desiccated coconut: Sprinkle over a bowl of berries and cream, or into curries.

Coconut water: Either buy a young, raw coconut and drain the water yourself, or buy coconut water in cartons. Check the label and make sure what you're buying is 100 per cent natural, with no added sugar or preservatives.

Coconut oil: This is one of the best oils for cooking with as it can withstand higher temperatures without being damaged like many oils. Buy a jar of 100 per cent organic, cold-pressed virgin coconut oil.

Coconut flour: A gluten-free alternative to traditional flour; it sucks up lots of water so you'll need to adapt your recipe when baking.

Coconut butter: Spread it on pancakes, use it in stir-fries or add a tablespoon to finish off a curry.

Coconut milk and cream: Perfect for curry sauces and desserts.

Raspberry coconut drink

For a refreshing coconut drink, blend 200 ml of coconut water with a handful of baby spinach and raspberries, plus the juice of half a lime.

2. Herbal teas

Many herbal teas have a slightly sweet flavour, which can be soothing if you're craving something comforting. Try the following:

Tea	Herbal tea	Fruit tea
Green tea	Rooibos tea	Cherry and cinnamon
Chai tea	Cardamom	Orange and coconut
Spiced black tea	Cinnamon	Mixed berry

	Ginger	Apple and ginger
	Vanilla	
	Chilli	
	Coconut	
	Roasted dandelion root	
	Peppermint or spearmint	
	Lavender	
	Hibiscus	
	Chamomile	
	Liquorice*	

*People suffering from hypertension should avoid excessive consumption

Note: Sadly, there's a proviso. If you regularly drink herbal teas containing fruit and citrus there is evidence this can strip away tooth enamel. Herbal teas with no fruit content, such as chamomile or peppermint, are not a danger to teeth. So use fruit teas occasionally and stick to herbal tea (or green tea, in limited amounts due to its caffeine content) for your daily consumption.

3. Spices

Spices such as cinnamon, nutmeg, cloves, cardamom and coriander can 'sweeten' food without adding sugar. Cinnamon in particular is a useful addition to your spice rack, as research suggests it reduces sugar cravings and stabilises blood sugar. Use at least half a teaspoon per meal or drink:

- Add to muesli or porridge
- Sprinkle over warm almond milk, coffee or smoothies
- Add to stewed or baked fruit
- Sprinkle over fruit and yoghurt desserts

4. Chocolate

The UK is a nation of chocoholics, but in a low-sugar/low-fructose diet, there's no place for super-sweet chocolate bars. Switch to dark chocolate, which contains less sugar and is rich in antioxidants.

Raw cacao powder or nibs (little bits)

Cacao is different to cocoa, which may be sitting in your kitchen cupboard as hot-chocolate powder. Raw cacao is made by cold-pressing unroasted cocoa beans so that the living enzymes stay in the bean and the fat (cocoa butter) is removed. Raw cacao is rich in minerals and potent antioxidants. It's also less than 1 per cent sugar. This gives you a clue as to how it tastes (it's pretty darn bitter). You can soften the taste by mixing it with other ingredients – see chocolate ideas below.

70-85 per cent cocoa dark chocolate

After raw cacao, the next best option is dark chocolate. Dark chocolate is rich in minerals such as iron and magnesium, but proceed with caution: it also has added fat and sugar. Look for a bar that is organic, free of additives, and ideally lists cocoa butter as the only fat. Stick to 70–85 per cent bars (85 per cent contains the least sugar) and savour just one or two squares at a time.

> *'I definitely get the occasional chocolate urge,*
> *but if it's good chocolate – over 70 per cent cocoa –*
> *one or two chunks sorts that out.'*
>
> Tom

Sugar-free chocolate?

Health food shops are overflowing with sugar-free chocolate. However, many bars are sweetened with agave, which is up to 90 per cent fructose, or maltitol which is a sugar alcohol that the body can't digest properly. Stick to raw cacao or 85 per cent dark chocolate.

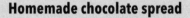

Homemade chocolate spread

Serves 1 (makes 2 tbsp)

Ingredients

- 1 tsp cacao powder
- 2 tbsp cashew butter
  (or other nut butter)

Instructions

Simply mix raw cacao powder with cashew nut butter to make the spread. Adjust the quantities to suit your taste.

DIY hot chocolate

Serves 1

Ingredients

- ½ can of coconut milk
- 1–2 tsp cacao powder
- ½ tsp of honey
- A dash of water
- Pinch of ground cinnamon

Instructions

Mix half a can of coconut milk with the cacao powder and heat in a saucepan until almost simmering. Add honey (or sweetener of your choice) for sweetness and a little water if the liquid is too thick or tastes too rich. Stir in a pinch or two of ground cinnamon.

Chocolate smoothie

Serves 1

Ingredients

- ½ can of coconut milk
- 1 banana
- 1 tbsp almond butter
- 1–2 tsp cacao powder

Instructions

Blend the banana with the almond butter, the cacao powder, and coconut milk. Add more or less coconut milk, depending on your preferred consistency.

5. Fruit

Yes, fruit contains fructose, but you'll also benefit from all the fibre, vitamins and minerals. Saying that, avoid eating the really sweet, high fructose fruits exclusively (see table in **Chapter 4**). Mix things up a bit. This makes sense from a nutrient point of view too – different fruits contain different nutrients.

Note: Given the choice of a piece of fruit or a standard chocolate bar, the fruit wins hands down in the health stakes. However, if you suffer from cravings, it's a good idea to focus on savoury snacks such as nuts over fruit, as sweet-tasting snacks can fuel sugar cravings. If you eat fruit between meals, eating it with something alkaline like a piece of cheese can help to protect your teeth (see box 'Why is it best to eat sweet things with meals?' later on in this chapter).

6. Sweet vegetables

Starchy vegetables – such as potatoes, sweet potatoes and butternut squash – raise blood sugar levels more than non-starchy vegetables, such as broccoli, cauliflower and green beans, but they contain important vitamins and minerals. Root vegetables are naturally sweet and are some of the most nutrient-dense vegetables you can eat. Just eat them in moderation.

Try eating more of these...

Sugar snap peas	Cherry tomatoes	Beetroot
Podded peas	Pumpkins	Butternut squash
Sweetcorn	Carrots	Sweet potatoes
Red peppers	Parsnips	Onions

> *'I have two bowls in the fridge – one with chopped veg and a light dressing, the other chopped fruits. A small bowl of either quietens the pangs.'*
> Cathi

7. Nuts

Nuts are highly nutritious and energy-dense, making them the perfect food to ward off cravings. Some nuts taste sweet and creamy, giving the illusion of having a sugary treat. Try raw macadamia and cashew nuts, and sweet-tasting nut butters.

Will nuts make me fat?

Numerous studies show that regular nut-eaters are more slender than those who shun nuts. They are also less likely to suffer from disease: the largest study ever conducted (Harvard School of Public Health's Nurses' Study of 127,000 women) found that people who ate a handful of nuts a day were 29 per cent less likely to die from heart disease and 11 per cent less likely to die from cancer over a 30-year period. Nuts are energy-dense and filling, making them an excellent choice for appetite control. They are rich in proteins, omega-3 fatty acids, antioxidants, vitamins and minerals.

Which nut is best?

The nurse's study couldn't determine if any one type of nut was better than any other, but it did find a link regarding how frequently nuts were eaten.

Those who ate nuts less than once a week had a 7 per cent reduction in mortality and those eating nuts seven or more times a week had a 20 per cent reduction in death rate.

How many nuts should I eat?

Have a small handful of nuts a day (around 30 g or an egg cupful). Eat a variety of different nuts, so you get a range of different nutrients – walnuts, Brazil nuts, almonds, hazelnuts, macadamias, pecans, pistachios, cashews and pine nuts. Peanuts are technically a legume and are best avoided or eaten in moderation as they are allergenic and can contain dangerous moulds that produce aflatoxin, a potent carcinogen.

8. Natural sweeteners

I lied when I said the eight foods in this chapter are naturally healthy and sweet. The sweeteners in this last section are sweet, but not necessarily healthy. Two natural sweeteners to consider are stevia and honey.

Stevia

Stevia is derived from the leaf of the stevia plant. It is around 300 times sweeter than table sugar, but it has negligible effects on blood sugar levels. It has virtually no calories and contains zero fructose, although some people complain certain brands have a bitter liquorice-like aftertaste. Most researchers say stevia is safe and there are claims that it lowers blood pressure and blood sugar levels. However, there are no long-term studies. As with artificial sweeteners, we don't know how the body responds to being primed for an influx of calories that never arrive.

Honey

Honey is another natural sweetener, which we discussed in detail in **Chapter 3**. It's 40 per cent fructose, so it's not something you want to spread thickly on your toast every morning. But raw, unprocessed honey does contain nutrients and enzymes.

Yacon and rice malt syrup

Some people recommend rice malt syrup and yacon. Both have pros and cons and there have been no long-term studies of either.

Brown rice syrup (also called rice malt syrup or rice syrup) is made from fermented cooked brown rice. On the plus side it's fructose-free, but on the downside it contains minimal nutrients and researchers have recently found high levels of arsenic in food flavoured with brown rice syrup. You'd probably have to be eating jars of the stuff for this to have an effect but it's your call. Yacon syrup is extracted from the roots of the yacon plant which grows in South America. It contains lots of fructooligosaccharides (FOS). These are sugar molecules that are connected in a way that makes them unrecognisable to the digestive system – so yacon syrup doesn't raise blood sugar levels. It is said to feed the friendly bacteria in the intestines, but it does contain a fair amount of fructose (though less than honey and agave).

In a nutshell, it's your call. Every sweetener has pros and cons. All sweeteners (natural and artificial) can keep you psychologically hooked on sugar. In the long term, the safest strategy is to use sweeteners in moderation or not at all. Savoury is the way to go!

Why is it best to eat sweet things with meals?

Experts believe that snacking between meals – whether you opt for junk or health food – is a major cause of weight gain and can interfere with the body's ability to burn fat. When we eat, our body releases insulin which helps carry sugar to our cells where it is used for energy. This sugar energy lasts for around 3 hours. After this our body switches to using energy from our fat stores. The bottom line: if we leave 4 to 5 hours between meals, we burn more fat.

In addition, snacking puts our liver and pancreas under stress and it's also bad for our teeth. When we eat sugary foods the sugar reacts with the bacteria in plaque (the sticky coating on your teeth) and produces harmful acids. Janet Clarke, from the British Dental Association, says: 'The more often we eat, the more frequently our teeth are attacked and are likely to decay. For this reason, I have an apple and an orange on my desk which I shall eat as part of my lunch, rather than a mid-afternoon snack.'

Chapter 6
Three Secret Weapons

There are three secret weapons when it comes to preventing cravings naturally. Combine all three strategies with a healthy low-sugar diet, and you'll be virtually bullet-proof.

1. Eat plenty of protein and healthy fats

Have you ever had this experience? You start a new healthy-eating regime and in a fit of enthusiasm you fix yourself an 'ultra-healthy' salad, consisting of nothing more than lettuce, cucumber, tomatoes and a drizzle of lemon juice dressing. But there's a problem. After polishing off your salad (in seconds), you feel ravenous and your eyes start to wander to the packet of chocolate-covered biscuits sitting on the sideboard…

If you eliminate sugary food from your diet **but don't replace it with nutritious and satisfying alternatives**, your body's stress response will kick in, cortisol levels will be raised, and you'll be overcome with an irresistible urge to find a quick source of energy (high-fat, high-sugar food) as soon as possible. The trick to successfully reducing your sugar intake is to never let your body feel it's being denied. The best way to do this is to eat 'logs' rather than 'twigs':

Eating sugary food and processed carbohydrates (e.g. white flour) is like putting dry twigs on an open fire – they flare up quickly but don't burn for long (i.e. you feel hungry soon after eating them). Fats and proteins, on the other hand, are like logs on your metabolic fire – they take longer to get going but they burn for hours. So, going back to our salad. If you add protein (some pieces of chicken, say) and fat (avocado and olives) to your dish, all of a sudden you have transformed your lacklustre and washed-out dish into a tasty, satisfying experience. Use this trick with every meal and you'll be amazed how quickly your cravings diminish.

Healthy fats: Avocados, butter, meat, oily fish, coconut and coconut oil, hemp oil, olives and olive oil, nut oils (unheated).

Healthy proteins: Eggs, nuts, cheese (cow, sheep or goat), full-fat yoghurt and Greek yoghurt, meat and poultry, fish and seafood.

Why fat is your friend

It's no wonder many people are scared to eat fat. For decades we've been told 'fat makes you fat'. But something's wrong. We have drastically cut the fat in our diet and obesity levels have rocketed. New research finds no evidence that saturated fat causes heart disease.* It's now suspected that the villain of the piece is actually sugar and refined carbohydrates. Unprocessed fats from meat, eggs, butter, avocado, nuts and coconut oil are vital for our health.

- Fats make us feel full and curb cravings.
- Fats enable the brain to function properly (the brain is mainly made of fat and cholesterol).

- Fats provide the building blocks for cell membranes and a variety of hormones.
- Fats act as carriers for important fat-soluble vitamins A, D, E and K.
- Fat raises levels of large, buoyant LDL cholesterol which can lower your risk of heart disease.

The fats to steer clear of are partially hydrogenated fats and trans fats. These are widely considered to be the worst type of fat you can eat as they are strongly linked with an increased risk of heart attack and stroke. They are created by heating and chemically treating vegetable and seed oils. You'll find them in margarines, processed food (biscuits, pies, cakes, ice cream, pastries) and fast food.

* Howard, B.V. et al., 'Low-Fat Dietary Pattern and Risk of Cardiovascular Disease: The Women's Health Initiative Randomised Controlled Dietary Modification Trial', *JAMA* 295 (2006): 655-66; Howard B.V. et al., 'Low Fat Dietary Pattern and Weight Change Over Seven Years: The Women's Health Initiative Dietary Modification Trial, *JAMA* 295 (2006): 39-49.

'Without even trying, by increasing the protein in my diet, I haven't eaten any chocolate for three days – which is the first time in ages.'
Sophie

2. Get enough sleep

You know when you have 'one too many' the night before and you wake up craving 'bad' food? Well, lack of sleep is like a mini hangover; it stresses the body and raises levels of cortisol*, which fuels our appetite and increases cravings, particularly for sugary and carb-laden treats. The brain feels the full brunt of this energy crisis. A recent study found that a single night of sleep deprivation not only increased people's desire for junk food, it also increased the pleasure they derived from eating these foods. And that was just a single night; not days, week or years of chronic poor sleep!

A single good night's sleep can restore your brain back to optimal function. But how much sleep is enough? Everyone has different needs, but 7–8 hours is about right for most people. According to Chinese medicine, our most regenerative sleep occurs between the hours of 11 p.m. and 1 a.m., so try to get to bed early in order to wake up feeling refreshed. You'll find further tips for getting a good night's sleep in **Chapter 14**.

*Cortisol increases the visceral fat we discussed in **Chapter 1**. The theory is that when our ancestors were stressed it was typically because they needed to run from a dangerous animal or fight off aggressive neighbours. Belly fat breaks down into fatty acids faster and these can zoom straight off to the liver for processing into energy. Back then, extra energy in the form of belly fat was a good thing. This is why chronic stress causes increased abdominal fat.

3. Exercise

Exercise really is your secret weapon when it comes to stabilising your blood sugar levels. Just 15 minutes on a treadmill has been shown to reduce cravings.

Exercise increases glucose metabolism and insulin sensitivity. After exercise, muscles refuel their glycogen stores by taking glucose from the bloodstream. To hurry this process along, they stimulate insulin receptors to increase their uptake of glucose and the body becomes more sensitive to insulin. More exercise means more muscle, and more muscle means better insulin sensitivity.

There's good stuff going on inside the brain too. When neuroscientists look inside the brains of new exercisers, they find an increased number of cells in the prefrontal cortex, the area of the brain involved in decision making. Exercise is an internal stress reducer, too. It lowers cortisol levels and releases feel-good endorphins. (It's as effective an antidepressant as Prozac and cognitive behavioural therapy.) There's even new evidence to suggest that exercise changes how we respond to the *idea* of food by reducing activation of the parts of the brain that are associated with food cravings.

> *'It's a vicious circle – overeating makes you sluggish and tired, and then exercise seems to be too much like hard work.'*
> Tom

If you've struggled to motivate yourself to exercise in the past, take heart. As you reduce your sugar intake your energy levels should increase and you'll have more 'oomph' to exercise.

One of the best ways to improve glucose metabolism is to include one or two high-intensity interval training sessions each week (see box).

High-intensity interval training (HIIT)

High-intensity interval training sounds daunting, but it simply involves exercising at high intensity interspersed with periods of moderate rest for between 4 and 20 minutes. A really quick HIIT session might involve 20 seconds of intensive activity followed by 10 seconds of rest. Repeat this for 4 minutes and you're done!

Aside from being one of the shortest workouts ever, the attraction of HIIT is that it improves glucose metabolism and fat burning. In a 2012 BBC *Horizon* documentary - *The Truth About Exercise* - Michael Mosley, a borderline diabetic, experienced a 24 per cent improvement in insulin sensitivity after four weeks of a 3 x 20-second HIIT regimen which he performed three times a week on an exercise bike.

Important note: If you're new to HIIT or exercise, please check with your doctor first before doing any intense training. Start by alternating a few minutes' brisk walking with recovery walking.

Part 3

RETRAIN YOUR BRAIN

Chapter 7

Be Kind to Yourself and Other Mind-bending Tips

Do you ever get the feeling there are two people living inside you? One person reacts to impulses and wants instant gratification ('Go on, have a piece of cheesecake, you've had a hard day'), while the other casts impulses aside and thinks long term ('Listen, you said you wanted to stop eating sugar; how's the cheesecake going to help?')? Some days the impulsive voice shouts louder and other days the wiser being gets heard. It often seems as if we are at the mercy of these two voices, with little or no control over what's going on.

Happily, you can train your brain to get better at self-control. The brain remodels itself based on what you ask it to do on a regular basis. Practise juggling every day and you get better at juggling. Practise worrying every day and your brain gets better at worrying. Practise a little self-control every day and your brain gets better at controlling your impulses.

If this sounds a little too simplistic, there is a proviso: as far as I know, there is no magic wand (read: willpower technique) that will obliterate sugar cravings while you continue to eat a high-sugar diet. However, if you take small steps to reduce your sugar intake AND use some of the strategies below, you should find your biological drive to eat sugar loosens its hold on you.

1. Ration your willpower

Dr Roy Baumeister is one of the leading experts in the field of willpower. His studies at Florida State University show that willpower has one central reserve. This explains why you're able to resist white toast and jam for breakfast, but after a long day making taxing decisions at work you come home and find it hard to resist opening a packet of crisps and a bottle of wine. Your willpower battery is running low. Controlling your temper, sticking to a budget, refusing second helpings, resisting cravings – these all tap into the same source. Trying to control too many aspects of your life is a strategy that can backfire badly. Choose your willpower challenges wisely and you won't deplete your willpower reserves.

2. Train your self-control muscle

What's the best thing to do if your willpower battery is running low? Answer: pick a tiny aspect of self-control and practise it every day. Like a muscle, self-control gets stronger through regular exercise. As it's a central reserve, other aspects of your life will start to benefit too.

In an Australian study, non-exercisers were encouraged to make use of a free gym membership. Most started cautiously with one session a week, but by the end of the two-month study, they were in the gym three times a week (note: starting small works!). The researchers were astounded to discover that this 'exercise treatment' increased self-control in *all* areas of the participants' lives. Without being asked to, they started smoking less, drinking less and consuming less caffeine. They were also spending less time watching TV and more time studying; they were saving more money and spending less on impulse purchases; and they were eating less junk food and more healthy food!

Choose one small aspect of self-control, practise it every day, and you should find other aspects of your life start clicking into place too. Small aspects of self-control around sugar include:

- Not eating boiled sweets in the car (eating nuts instead)
- Writing one line in your food diary each night
- Making your second glass of wine a spritzer
- Going for a 5-minute walk rather than drinking a sugary fizzy drink

3. Beware the 'what-the-hell' effect

Sometimes things go wrong. Let's say you have a bad day and eat a packet of digestive biscuits. You then feel so bad and consumed with guilt that you forget all the successful small steps you've taken up to this point and plunge into a vortex of overeating. Researchers describe this as the 'what-the-hell' effect. 'What the hell; I've had a bite of cake now, I may as well finish the rest of it.' If this sounds familiar, there's something you can do to help break the cycle…

4. Be kind to yourself

Psychologists studying the what-the-hell effect have discovered it doesn't work in quite the way we expect. In an American study, two groups of women were given a doughnut to eat and were then asked to help themselves to as many sweets as they wanted. One group of women received a message about self-compassion after eating the doughnut, the other group received no message. Guess who ate the most sweets? Women who were encouraged to forgive themselves ate 28 g of sweets, whereas the women who received no message about self-compassion ate 70 g of sweets on average!

This seems to fly in the face of everything we know about striving to achieve our goals. The key to success, we believe, is to be really hard on ourselves. Research shows this creates **less** motivation and **worse** self-control, because it drives the brain into reward-seeking mode (i.e. we turn to sweet things to make ourselves feel better). The next time you suffer a temporary setback, talk to yourself as you would talk to your best friend, and offer support and encouragement. Your setback doesn't mean anything other than the fact that you are human. Your aim is to look after your health: big congratulations are in order! You are allowed to falter. You don't have to be perfect. All that matters is that you pick yourself up and keep going.

5. Know why you're doing this (and polish your crystal ball)

The part of the brain that you're recruiting when you're able to resist impulses and cravings is the prefrontal cortex; a chunk of brain right behind your forehead. Its job is to steer us towards doing the right thing so that we achieve our goals. When you start eyeing up the dessert menu in a restaurant, the prefrontal cortex reminds you that your goal is to stop eating so much sugar, so you'd better order coffee instead.

You can give your prefrontal cortex a helping hand by formulating a clear statement of intent. Knowing what you want and why you want it will make it much easier to say 'no' to the things that won't help you achieve your goal and 'yes' to the things that will ensure your success.

To help you clarify a statement of intent around sugar, imagine how things will look in the future when your willpower is firing on all cylinders.

- How will you benefit from reducing sugar in your diet?
- How will your life change?
- Who else will benefit?
- How will you feel about yourself as you keep taking small steps and move towards your goal?

6. Why stress is the enemy of willpower (and what to do about it)

The reason it's harder to resist temptation when you're feeling stressed is because the fight-or-flight response takes over. Stress hormones are released from your adrenal glands and every cell in your body is alert and primed for action – every cell, that is, apart from your brain. The logical-thinking prefrontal cortex is shut down and your impulses take over – so that you don't spend ages thinking about what to do in an emergency, and instinctively do something useful, like fight or run for your life. Research shows when cortisol floods the bloodstream, it increases caloric intake of 'comfort foods'. Stress is a part of our everyday lives, so what's the solution?

Pause...

The fight-or-flight response works to speed you up. The antidote is to slow down your breathing. This turns on the relaxation (parasympathetic) response and activates your prefrontal cortex, giving it a chance to jump in and help you to make the right choice. Spend 10–15 seconds taking one full in-and-out breath (do this gently and don't force it). Breathe in through your nose, purse your lips and breathe out slowly through your mouth.

Extending your exhalation like this is the easiest way to slow down your breathing. Do this for a minute or two and you'll feel calmer and more in control. Pausing like this takes us off autopilot. We realise we have a choice. There's no universal rule that says we have to do what our impulses order. We can ignore our impulses and choose something better.

Warning: Don't deploy this technique for the first time when you're staring down a chocolate bar! Practise it from time to time during the day and it will be easier to switch to it when you need to.

'I eat more sugary things when I'm bored or stressed. When I'm not at work I will be able to go for days without even thinking about snacking.'
Jason

'I'm a big emotional eater – I tend to eat sugary treats when I'm bored and stressed. I call it "entertainment eating".'
Ali

'I love pain au raisin and cinnamon swirls. The crazy thing is that I don't have these regularly unless I tell myself I need to cut down on sugar!'
Rachael

> 'I am very much an emotional eater. I celebrate with sugary foods and drinks, such as cakes, doughnuts, fizzy drinks, especially on birthdays, anniversaries, promotions etc. When feeling down or stressed, I turn to comfort food such as biscuits.'
> Zeba

7. Replace eating with a feel-good behaviour

According to American Psychological Association (APA) surveys, only 16 per cent of people who eat to reduce stress say that it helps them. In studies, women were more likely than men to turn to chocolate when they felt anxious or depressed, but the only reliable mood change they experienced was an increase in feelings of guilt! The APA suggests we should ditch food and drink as feel-good strategies and turn to feel-good behaviours instead. Strategies that are most effective at making us feel better include:

- Going for a walk
- Spending time on a creative hobby
- Exercising and playing sport
- Meditating or practising yoga
- Praying or attending a religious service
- Reading
- Listening to music

- Spending time with friends or family
- Having a massage

These activities trigger the release of feel-good brain chemicals such as serotonin and oxytocin in the brain. Because these activities soothe the brain and body rather than excite it, it can be easy to overlook them and forget how good they make us feel.

Chapter 8
Breaking Habits

'Retirement brought another meal into my day – 4 p.m. afternoon tea with a scone and jam! So at a time when I have more time for exercise and planning our food, I'm adding a risk. How crazy is that?'
Cathi

'My worst habit is eating cakes and puddings when I eat out with friends.'
Anna

'When I'm working late on the computer and my energy levels are really low, I start snacking.'
Sophie

When was the last time you opened a bottle of wine and thought, 'Mmm, I'll just have some celery and hummus to go with that'? Whether it's alcohol and crisps, or a cup of tea and a slice of cake, habits underlie much of our sugar addiction.

This is how habits are formed: let's say you reward yourself with a bar of chocolate while watching TV when you come home from work. Over time, your brain learns to associate the pleasure you get from watching TV with the pleasure (dopamine hit) of eating chocolate. The two go hand in hand. So watching TV becomes a habit that triggers eating chocolate. It can get to the point where you don't feel able to relax in front of the TV unless you have chocolate (or wine or sweets, or whatever your favourite 'treat' is).

Just as we can make habits, we can break them. Brain scans show that structural changes occur in the brain throughout our lives. New neurons, and fresh connections between neurons, are constantly being made. This 'neuroplasticity' is great news. It means that, with practice, we can create new neural pathways that endorse healthier eating habits.

Step 1: Notice when you give in to temptation

The first step to breaking a sugar habit is learning how and when you give in to temptation. Chances are you don't eat cakes or crisps 24/7. Sometimes you can resist the urge and sometimes you can't. For the next day or two, simply notice what's going on. The second you realise you're about to give in to a craving for sugar, get curious. What's the situation? What's the environment? Who's with you? What are you thinking or saying to yourself that makes it more likely you'll give in to temptation? Does being worried or tired or overworked affect your choices? Notice when stress strikes, either at home or at work, and what happens to your self-control. Try to catch yourself earlier and earlier in this process.

It's also useful to take note of whether certain decisions helped or hindered your willpower. Did you get up early and make a packed lunch so you wouldn't be tempted to eat something 'bad' in the canteen? Did you get caught up in a phone call at work, leave work late and pick up a takeaway on the way home because you wouldn't have time to cook?

The next time you're tempted, turn your attention inward.

Step 2: List your sugar habits

Knowing when your willpower falters is crucial information because it means you can start to avoid the traps and triggers that herald an impending willpower meltdown. Start by making a list of all your sugar-eating habits. It's important to focus on the daily habits first, not the ones you do once a month or so. It might help to think about different situations. For example:

Environments
- Cinema + caramel popcorn
- Service station + hot chocolate or sugary coffee
- Train station + chocolate muffin

Activities
- Shopping + cake
- TV + chocolate
- Exercise + sports drink

People
- Work colleagues + birthday treats
- Best friend + ice cream
- Partner + takeaway

Physical sensations

- Afternoon slump + sugar in tea
- Stressed + wine
- Bored + biscuits

Times of day

- 11 a.m. + cereal bar
- 6 p.m. + alcohol

Food and drink

- Tea + sugar
- Wine + nibbles
- Coffee + biscuit
- Breakfast + fruit juice
- Fast-food burger + soft drink
- Gin + tonic

Step 3: Plan ahead

Once you've listed your habits, there are several ways you begin to break their spell:

1. You can avoid the thing that triggers your habit.
2. You can replace your response to the trigger with a sugar-free alternative.
3. You can put an obstacle in the way of you and temptation.

All three strategies will require some planning and preparation. You need to be clear as to exactly how you're going to deal with specific sugar habits, so that you're ready to act when they crop up again in the future.

Strategy 1: Avoid the trigger

An obvious solution is to simply avoid the events associated with eating sugar altogether. OK, you can't cancel Christmas or ostracise your best friend. This won't work on every habit. Here are some ideas:

- Drive a different route back from work and avoid the service station.
- Walk a different route and avoid the vending machine/coffee shop.
- Shop with friends who support or share your low-sugar goals (and don't want to stop for coffee and cake).
- Avoid the kitchen at work when you know someone's bought cakes in – just don't go there!
- Switch to a different local café that sells healthy low-sugar foods.

Strategy 2: Change your response

This strategy involves keeping the habit (watching TV) but swapping your response (eating chocolate) for a sugar-free alternative. Make sure you have the alternative immediately to hand. You want to make it as easy as possible to switch. For example:

- When watching TV, have healthy snacks nearby, such as vegetable crudités or kale and sweet potato crisps (see **Chapter 12**).
- Replace the box of biscuits sitting next to the kettle with a jar of nuts and seeds.

- If you make a gin and tonic, swap the tonic for soda water with a squeeze of lemon.
- After finishing a project, give yourself a non-food reward such as watching a favourite DVD.
- Cut down on takeaways and make Friday night 'homemade curry night', using fresh ingredients.
- Swap your burger and fizzy drink for a burger and bottle of sparkling water.

Strategy 3: Create an obstacle

Two factors make it much more likely that you'll give in to a sugar habit. **The temptation must be available immediately** *and* **you need to see it**. If the treat is out of sight and far away, this makes the treat more abstract and less exciting to the brain. Delaying the gratification in this way gives your rational mind (prefrontal cortex) a chance to kick in and override your impulse.

Little tricks work well: one study found that simply placing sweets in an opaque jar on office workers' desks rather than a clear jar, reduced consumption by a third. When the jars were placed 6 feet away, so people had to get up to grab the sweets, consumption dropped by another third. Knowing this, you can tweak your environment in order to reduce temptation:

- Don't leave sugary snacks where you can see them. Out of sight is out of mind.
- Move temptations as far away from you as possible so you have to make an effort to get them.

- Get rid of temptation by removing all sugary snacks and drinks from your house or office space.

Another trick is to implement a 10-minute delay. If you feel the urge to eat something sweet, like a Danish pastry for example, tell yourself you can have the pastry, but you need to wait 10 minutes first. Move yourself away from the treat if possible, so that the reward seems less appealing to the brain. Once the 10 minutes are up, if you still want to eat the pastry, spend some time reflecting on your statement of intent and the long-term reward you will gain by not eating the pastry (see **Chapter 7**). If you still want to eat the pastry, go ahead. By sticking to a 10-minute delay, you will be building your self-image as someone who can resist temptation and strengthening your ability to say no. (Tip: try drinking a glass of water during your 10-minute delay. It's a good distraction technique and, after a quick hydration fix, you may feel less tempted to indulge in sugar.)

Celebrate each time you stick to your guns; you are building new neural networks in your brain which will make it easier and easier to resist temptation as time passes. These new neural networks won't spring up overnight. The key to creating 'I don't need sugar' pathways in your brain is repetition. Keep at it and things will get easier!

Chapter 9
Happy Eating

There's one diet that stands head and shoulders above all the rest. It doesn't cost any money. It doesn't require you to starve yourself. And it can gently and naturally wean you off sugar. Some have called it 'the greatest diet in the world'. (This had better be good.) Here it is:

Eat when you are hungry, choose the foods your body is hungry for and stop before you're too full.

It sounds simple, but how the heck do you do this? A growing body of research suggests 'mindful eating' could be the answer. Think back over the past few days. How often did you eat your food on 'autopilot'? Were there times when you sat down in front of the TV with your supper on your lap and looked down a few minutes later to discover, with a shock, that your plate was empty and you still felt hungry? Have you ever devoured a chocolate bar or drained a third glass of wine and realised afterwards that you didn't really want it, or that the very thing you thought would make you feel better, has actually made you feel *worse*?

Mindful eating is based on the Buddhist concept of mindfulness, which involves focusing your attention on the present moment. I call it 'happy eating' because it's about making eating more pleasurable and satisfying. (It's also one of the fastest relaxation techniques I know.) It entails taking ourselves off 'autopilot'; tasting our food, perhaps for the first time in years, and noticing how different foods affect our body and emotions. Whether you turn to 'treats' whenever you feel stressed, reach for the biscuit jar out of habit at 11 a.m., or eat piles of food but somehow never quite feel satisfied, mindful eating can steer you towards healthier food choices and behaviours and help put you back in control of your sugar intake.

Mindfulness and meditation research

Research into mindful eating is still in its infancy, but so far research shows it reduces cravings and episodes of binge eating. Regular meditation can also help. Meditation alters brain activity and structure in several beneficial ways:

- It increases blood flow to the part of the brain (the insula) associated with awareness of bodily sensations, such as feeling full.[1] Meditators have a thicker anterior insula.

- It increases the activity of the area of the brain responsible for decision-making (the dorsolateral prefrontal cortex), making it easier to make healthier food choices.[2]

- It increases blood flow to the self-control hub of the brain (the anterior cingulate cortex), which helps us deal with impulses such as food cravings.[3]

Six keys to mindful eating

There are six keys to mindful eating but you don't have to implement all of them in one go! Pick one or two tips that appeal to you, give them a go and see what happens.

1. Eat when you're genuinely hungry

Every day we rely on a host of external cues to tell us when to eat. We eat because other people are eating, because 'it's time to eat', because we've completed an onerous task and are due a 'reward', or simply because we're angry, lonely or bored. To tap back into your internal hunger cues, try the following:

- Ask yourself how hungry you are on a scale of one to ten. Genuine hunger is roughly seven on this scale.
- Check whether you're open to options. When people use food for comfort, they tend to crave a particular type of food (ice cream, chocolate, pizza) and only that food will do. In contrast, when we're genuinely hungry, we're more open to options.
- Tiredness can be a sign of dehydration. If you haven't had anything to drink for a while, drink a glass of water and wait for 10 minutes to see if you still feel hungry.

> *'I usually crave cream cakes although after eating them I feel a little down. While I'm in the midst of my rabid craving state, I know that only cakes can satisfy me.'*
>
> Ali

2. Eat what your body needs

Studies show the brain lights up in anticipation of a reward. So the mere sight of a pastry or the smell of a baked cake can trigger the brain to release dopamine. Before we know it, we're speed-walking to the nearest shop (or our kitchen cupboard) for a sugar fix. Pausing for a few seconds can make a massive difference to your food choice:

1. To avoid being swayed by external cues tempting you to eat certain foods, tune in to your body. Imagine you're having a chat with your stomach. Does it need something sweet or savoury, crunchy or smooth, light or filling?
2. Picture some foods that fit this description.
3. Imagine their taste, texture, and smell and most importantly, *how you'll feel once you've eaten them.*
4. Keep 'trying on' different foods in this way until you hit on something that feels perfect for your stomach.

If your stomach ignores you or tells you it 'needs' a double-chocolate-chip muffin, don't despair. As you keep practising the techniques in this chapter, you'll find it easier and easier to tune in to your body and differentiate 'needs' from 'wants'.

3. Eat slowly

It can take around 20 minutes for your brain to receive the message that your stomach is full. If you bolt your food in 5 minutes, the 'I'm full' message will arrive too late – by this time you may have helped yourself to seconds or be reaching for a dessert. Using a trigger to relax when you eat can help to slow down your eating:

- Take one full breath in through your nose and breathe out s-l-o-w-l-y through your mouth.
- Inhale, shrug your shoulders up towards your ears and exhale as you let your shoulders gently drop.
- Repeat the phrase 'soft belly' and let the tension melt away from your stomach.

Tips on becoming a slow eater:

- Chew each mouthful fully – until the food has lost all its texture. Chewing also improves digestion, so helping your body absorb more nutrients.
- Eat with your non-dominant hand.
- Use a small fork or a teaspoon. (This is not something you'll want to do forever, but it's a good way of breaking the habit of taking large mouthfuls of food.)
- Set a kitchen timer to 20 minutes and see if you can take this long to eat your meal.
- Place a little note where you eat ('pause', 'slow' or 'relax') to remind you to slow down.

Why does it take 20 minutes for us to feel full?

The reason we feel full is because stretch receptors in the stomach are activated as the stomach fills with food. Hormones – such as peptide YY (PYY) and cholecystokinin (CCK) – are also released when food is detected in the small intestine. It takes roughly 20 minutes for food to move from the stomach to the small intestine.

4. Focus on your food

If our minds are distracted, we miss out on the taste, texture and smell of food, all of which contribute to feelings of satiety. This is particularly important when eating sugary food. The next time you eat a dessert or some dark chocolate try focusing 100 per cent on the experience. You should find, with practice, you need to eat less before feeling satisfied. The following tips can help:

- Eat your meals away from any distractions – TV, mobile, computer.

- Before you start to eat, really *look* at your food – all the colours, shapes and textures.

- Notice any feelings of impatience – any habitual urges to rush your food.

- While eating, see how many flavours and textures you can detect.

- Don't forget to use your other senses – the smell of fresh basil, the crunch as you bite into a carrot.

- Monitor how different foods 'sit' in your stomach. Which foods make you feel alert and energetic? Which foods make you feel bloated, uncomfortable or sleepy?

- Notice how you feel an hour or so after eating. How's your energy? How does your stomach feel? How's your mood?

'The first time I ate a meal mindfully, I realised I hadn't really "eaten" in years. I used to eat "and" – the "and" could be reading, watching TV or answering emails.'

Karen

Mini food or drink meditation

You can do this mini meditation in a crowded café or while sitting at your desk, without anyone noticing. The aim is to achieve a 30-second burst of high-intensity mindfulness. Try using this technique while taking the first bite of a peach or the first sip of herbal tea.

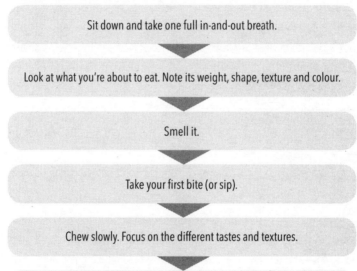

Sit down and take one full in-and-out breath.

Look at what you're about to eat. Note its weight, shape, texture and colour.

Smell it.

Take your first bite (or sip).

Chew slowly. Focus on the different tastes and textures.

Swallow the mouthful. (End of meditation.)

Notice how relaxed you feel and how still your mind has become.

5. Eat until you are satiated (not stuffed)

Eat until you feel satisfied, but not 100 per cent full (or 'stuffed', to use a technical term). Many cultures have a tradition of eating like this. In Japan, the advice is to stop eating when you are 80 per cent full; in India, the Ayurvedic tradition advises eating until you are 75 per cent full; the Chinese specify 70 per cent. The precise figures don't matter; the main thing is to put down your knife and fork before you are 100 per cent full. (You can take your pick and visualise this as being anything between 70–80 per cent.)

- When nearing the end of a meal, focus on your stomach and gauge how full you feel on a scale of one to ten. Stop eating when you reach seven.

- When the French finish a meal, they don't say 'I'm full', they say *Je n'ai plus faim* – 'I have no more hunger'. Stop eating **when you no longer have hunger**, rather than when you are full.

- Try using smaller plates and bowls. Food served on a small plate looks larger than the same portion served on a larger plate, so we feel more satisfied. Ditto for your wine or beer glasses – a tall, thin glass looks as if it contains more than a short, wide glass.

- If you feel the urge for a second helping, remember the 20-minute rule. Move away from the table and wait for a few minutes. This is easier to do if you've savoured your food.

6. Keep track of positive changes

As you practise mindful eating, you'll notice your relationship with food is changing. It's important to note (and celebrate) these changes in order to positively reinforce your new way of eating. This needn't be anything formal – make a mental note to yourself, share what you're discovering with friends or keep a journal and write a few words every day.

Here's a little quiz to help you get a feeling for how you're doing:

- Are you noticing how different foods make you feel?
- Are you tuning in to whether you're hungry, thirsty or bored?
- Are you slowing down and tasting your food more?
- Has eating become more pleasurable?
- How quickly do you feel satiated?
- Is it getting easier to make healthier food choices?
- Are your cravings going?

A final word on perseverance

Many of us are used to being entertained while we eat (by the TV or Internet, etc.), so it can be a struggle to switch to being 'entertained' by our food alone. There will be times when you manage to focus 100 per cent and your experience of eating will be totally transformed. But equally, there will be times when it feels like mindful eating is just about the most boring thing in the world!

This is all totally normal. Don't panic or beat yourself up. Keep gently bringing your attention back to chewing and tasting your food. If you persevere, you'll be amazed at how pleasurable and relaxing eating becomes, and how much more confidence you have in your ability to tune in to what your body needs and walk away from sugary food.

Don't be concerned if you practise for a few days and then forget. When you realise you've stopped using the techniques, just pick up where you left off. None of the techniques are difficult; the trickiest thing is remembering to use them!

Important note: The aim of this chapter is to help you learn to trust your body's signals, as opposed to reducing your appetite or suppressing your body's signals to eat. If you have any concerns about the amount you're eating or you feel that your focus on food intake is becoming too overpowering, please seek help: Beat provides helplines, online support and a network of UK-wide self-help groups to help adults and young people in the UK beat their eating disorders www.b-eat.co.uk).

[1.] 'Meditation experience is associated with increased cortical thickness', *NeuroReport* (2005) vol. 16, no. 17: 1893–1897.

[2.] 'The measurement of regional cerebral blood flow during the complex cognitive task of meditation: a preliminary SPECT study', *Psychiatry Research: Neuroimaging* (2001) vol. 106, no. 2: 113–122.

[3.] 'Mechanisms of white matter changes induced by meditation', *Proceedings of the National Academy of Sciences of the United States of America* (2012) vol. 109, no. 26.

Part 4

A LOW-SUGAR DAY

Chapter 10
Breakfast

> *'I used to eat cereal for breakfast – a huge bowl – and by 10 a.m. I was starving!'*
>
> Katie

Mornings can be a sugar minefield. With long commutes, early meetings and kids' school runs, our biggest concern is time rather than nutrition: 'What can I eat that can be prepared in seconds?' Add feeling tired or stressed into the equation, and our ability to make good food choices may be at an all-time low. Even if we opt for the 'healthy' option (muesli, fruit and orange juice, anyone?), it's likely that by mid-morning we'll start feeling peckish and crave a sweet-tasting pick-me-up. Sugar lurks in the most unexpected breakfast foods – even the supposedly healthy ones.

Sugar traps

As with all of the following meal chapters, we'll get the bad news out of the way first by looking at where hidden sugar lurks in our breakfast foods before moving on to the good news – quick, delicious alternatives that will help you start your day in a sugar-free way.

Table sugar

An obvious source of sugar in the morning is the granulated stuff you add to your tea, coffee, porridge or cereal. You may be only adding a teaspoon here or there, but it soon adds up. Two cups of tea with a teaspoon of sugar in each, another sprinkled over your breakfast cereal, plus the 5 or so teaspoons hiding *in* your cereal… you could easily have eaten 8 teaspoons of sugar before stepping out of the house!

Cereals

The sugar content of shop-bought cereals often takes people by surprise. It goes without saying that chocolate cereals are high in sugar, e.g., Tesco Choco Snaps (35 per cent sugar) and Sainsbury's Choco Rice Pops (also 35 per cent). However, the figures for non-chocolate cereals are equally as shocking, e.g. Kellogg's Ricicles (40 per cent) and Honey Monster Sugar Puffs (31 per cent). Even so-called 'healthy' cereals contain more sugar per serving than a jam doughnut*:

The sugar content of 'healthy' breakfast cereals

Cereal	Sugar content
Dorset Cereals Luscious Berries & Cherries	36 per cent sugar (4 tsp per 45 g serving)
Alpen Original Muesli	23 per cent sugar (2½ tsp per 45 g serving)
Kellogg's All-Bran Flakes	20 per cent sugar (2 tsp per 45 g serving)
Kellogg's Special K	17 per cent sugar (just under 2 tsp per 45 g serving)
Dorset Cereals Simply Delicious Muesli	17 per cent sugar (just under 2 tsp per 45 g serving)

* A jam doughnut is typically 10–15 per cent sugar (approx. 2 teaspoons per doughnut)

When looking at these figures, bear in mind that the suggested serving size on most cereals is a miniscule 30–45 g. This makes the sugar 'per serving' figure look more reasonable. The reality is, many of us pour ourselves a serving several times the size of this (try weighing out 30 g of your favourite cereal and you'll see what I mean).

Watch out for these other clever marketing ploys:

- Cereals that are marketed as being 'high in fibre' and low in fat' are often flakes coated in honey or sugar, mixed with dried fruit. (I hereby rename them 'Fructose Flakes'.)

- Phrases such as 'sweetened with honey', 'no added sugar' and 'natural sugars' are code for 'contains fructose'. Honey is 40 per cent fructose. Dried fruit is almost 70 per cent sugar, a large proportion of which is fructose.

- Roasted and toasted cereals, such as granola, have extra sugar added to aid in the toasting. Many are 20 per cent sugar.

Low-sugar cereals

If you want to avoid the sugar traps, switch to low-sugar cereals such as **shredded wheat**, **wheat biscuits** or **sugar-free dried-fruit-free muesli**. This small change can cut your sugar intake in one fell swoop. A 30 g serving of bran flakes can contain up to 2.4 teaspoons of sugar (assuming, of course, you stick to the 30 g). A serving of two wheat biscuits contains under half a teaspoon of sugar. Do this every day and you'll slash your weekly sugar consumption by 14 teaspoons! The best option of all is to **make your own muesli** – it takes seconds to make, you control the ingredients, and it will store in an airtight container for several months (see the recipe at end of this chapter). For a warm, comforting breakfast, serve your homemade muesli with warmed milk.

Bread

I'm afraid there's more bad news about bread (I know; I wasn't happy about it either). Many shop-bought breads contain a surprising amount of sugar. Traditionally, white bread (4 per cent) and bagels (6.5 per cent) were the worst offenders, but recent analysis of some brown and wholemeal brands has revealed many contain more added sugar than their supposedly inferior cousins, with some individual slices containing more than half a teaspoon of total sugars. Manufacturers say it's to 'mask' the bitter taste of wholemeal flour and the amount of sugar added is 'negligible' – but, as we know, it all adds up.

There's an additional reason why bread is not your friend. As most of the nutritious part of the grain is removed in the milling process, all types of bread are rapidly converted to sugar once digested – even wholegrain varieties! The same goes for breakfast cereals.

Low-sugar bread

Sourdough bread tends to contain less sugar and it's made with a naturally occurring bacteria which produces a lower glucose and insulin response than bread leavened with regular baker's yeast. **Rye** bread and **wholemeal pitta** breads are also good options. When baking bread at home, try using coconut flour which doesn't cause strong sugar spikes. Making your own bread puts you firmly in control of your sugar intake.

Spreads

Many jams and spreads are over 50 per cent sugar – you may as well spread a chocolate bar on your toast!*

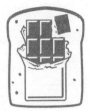

Sugar content of jams and spreads

Spread	Sugar content
Honey	78–83 per cent
Jams and conserves	50–70 per cent
Hazelnut spreads	50–55 per cent
Lemon or orange curd	46–51 per cent
Marshmallow Fluff	49 per cent

* A bar of milk chocolate is around 50 per cent sugar

Low-sugar spreads

Your best bet is to go for **nut butters** such as cashew, almond or hazelnut (you'll find them in health shops and large supermarkets) or **coconut butter**. **Yeast extract spreads** contain minimal or no sugar, but they contain high levels of salt, so spread thinly. **Organic peanut butter** is usually 2–3 per cent sugar. Buy organic as these products are less likely to contain pesticides, fungus and aflatoxin, a potent carcinogenic mould which can grow on peanuts (yum). If you love peanut butter, it's probably best to eat it in moderation (rather than spoonfuls every day). Or go totally natural and mash half an **avocado** with some black pepper and lemon juice and spread this on your toast.

Fruit juice

When pouring your next glass of juice, there is one cheery little fact you need to know: **a glass of juice contains as much sugar as a glass of Coke!**

It doesn't matter whether the juice is organic, freshly squeezed in a café, out of a carton, or you have juiced it yourself at home. A 330 ml can of cola and a 330 ml serving of apple juice both contain around 8 teaspoons of sugar. Remember, juices are particularly hazardous to health. As the sugar is in liquid form with no fibre, the sugar reaches the liver faster. The liver struggles to cope with this and converts much of this sugar to fat.

Follow these fruity guidelines:

- Eat your fruit whole.
- Swap your juicer for a blender, so you eat the whole fruit. (I have heard blending fruit destroys the fibre, but I couldn't find studies. Whichever way you look at it, a smoothie still contains some fibre, so it's not as bad as a juice.)
- Focus on vegetable smoothies that contain one piece of fruit for sweetness.
- If you do drink the odd glass of juice, stick to low-sugar juices such as grapefruit, dilute your juice with water, and avoid high-sugar juices such as grape.

A quick word about milk

Plain milk doesn't contain sucrose or fructose, so it's not a 'high-sugar' food. However, the jury is out on whether milk is suitable for regular human consumption. It's estimated that around 5 per cent of the population in Britain suffer from lactose intolerance. In addition, many experts argue that the pasteurisation process destroys milk's enzymes, vitamins and proteins, and that milk can stimulate insulin production. (It is thought this is due to the special combination of lactose and protein that's found in milk.)

If you drink milk, buy **organic whole milk** if possible. 'Organic' so that it's hormone- and antibiotic-free; 'whole' because it's the cream that contains the fat-soluble vitamins A, D, E and K. Semi-skimmed and skimmed milk are less nutritious and tend to contain more lactose (lactose is found in the water-based portion of milk).

Alternatively, switch to (unsweetened) **coconut milk**, **almond milk**, **oat milk** or **rice milk**. There is some concern about the safety of soya and soy products, as some research has shown that the phytoestrogens in soy beans promote breast cancer growth in animals.

Low- or no-sugar breakfasts

If you've been eating the same breakfast every day for years, it can be hard to imagine an alternative exists. But it does – your taste buds just don't know it yet. The number one thing to concentrate on at breakfast time (actually, at *all* mealtimes) is eating some protein and fat. This will provide your body with a slow-burning fuel that will keep you energised for hours – which means fewer cravings for sugar and less of an urge to snack later on.

Good sources of fat	Good sources of protein
Avocados	Eggs*
Butter	Nuts
Meat**	Cheese (cow, sheep or goat)
Coconut and coconut oil	Full-fat yoghurt & Greek yoghurt
Olives and olive oil	Meat and poultry**
Nut oils (unheated)	Fish and seafood (e.g. wild salmon and tuna)
Hemp oil	
Oily fish (salmon, mackerel, sardines, trout, herring, anchovies)	

* It's a misconception that eggs are linked to high cholesterol levels and heart disease. They contain high-quality proteins, fats, vitamins and minerals and are one of healthiest and most complete natural foods you can eat. There is no recommended limit for how many we should eat, so don't be afraid to eat eggs several times a week.

** Sausages, bacon, ham and other processed meats contain salt and preservatives, such as sodium nitrite, which have been linked with cancer and heart disease. To limit your risk, avoid consuming these foods on a daily basis and, wherever possible, choose good quality, fresh meat over packaged, processed products.

Low-sugar breakfast ideas

Cereal

Homemade muesli (see recipe)

A handful of berries with nuts, yoghurt and coconut flakes

Shop-bought sugar-free, dried-fruit-free muesli

Wheat biscuits (unflavoured)

Shredded wheat (unflavoured)

Porridge mixed with cinnamon and topped with berries

Toast

Toasted sourdough or rye bread topped with…

- Nut butter, organic peanut butter or yeast extract spread
- ½ a mashed avocado with leftover roasted vegetables and a drizzle of olive oil
- Cheese and sliced tomato with black pepper and dried basil (under the grill)
- Mashed avocado with Parma ham or sliced strawberry and goats' cheese (under the grill)

Fruit

Fruit salad with macadamia cream and flaked almonds

Coconut flour pancakes with berries and macadamia cream

Vegetable and fruit smoothies (see recipe later on in the chapter)

Cooked breakfast

Poached egg and wilted spinach on sourdough toast with a knob of butter

Poached egg on Swiss chard sautéed with garlic and topped with grated parmesan

Boiled egg with steamed asparagus soldiers or a little sea salt

Scrambled egg, feta and spinach (see recipe later on in the chapter)

Scrambled egg with smoked salmon and half an avocado

Mushroom omelette with avocado, tomato and coriander salad

Spinach and goat's cheese omelette topped with sliced avocado

Bacon, eggs, grilled tomatoes and mushrooms

Hash made with leftover vegetables plus egg, cheese, fresh herbs and/or leftover fish or meat

Note: A 1-tablespoon serving of tomato sauce contains 1 teaspoon of sugar! Make your own homemade tomato sauce or switch to mustard.

Mindfulness reminder

Breakfast is the time of day we are most likely to bolt down our food as we rush to leave the house. This is the perfect time to practise mindful eating technique 3 (eat slowly) from **Chapter 9**. Try putting a little note or object on the breakfast table to remind you of your relaxation trigger and the need to slow down (have fun with this; it could be any object that has meaning for you).

Habit reminder

To avoid rushing in the morning, get your breakfast ingredients ready the night before – put them on the kitchen counter or group them in the fridge so it's easy to grab everything in the morning. Prepare as much as you can the night before. Try putting a few tablespoons of yoghurt in a glass jar with a piece of chopped fruit or a handful of berries. Add nuts, seeds and coconut flakes in the morning… breakfast in 5 seconds!

Exercise reminder

Yoga and meditation are a great way to ease you into the day and will help you to leave the house feeling calm. Follow a 20-minute yoga DVD (see **Resources** chapter at the end of this book) or sign up to an online yoga class of your choice at YogaGlo.com. Researchers at the University of Bristol have found that employees who exercise before going to work are happier and better equipped to handle whatever the day throws at them.

Breakfast recipes

Feta and Spinach Scrambled Egg

(serves 2)

Ingredients

- 5 medium eggs
- 2–3 handfuls of spinach
- 100 g of cubed feta
- Knob of butter or coconut oil

Instructions

Wash the spinach and cook for 2–3 minutes in a saucepan until wilted, then drain. (There's no need for oil as the spinach will steam in the water left on the leaves.) While the spinach is cooking, beat the eggs in a bowl and add black pepper. Melt a knob of butter or coconut oil, add the eggs and stir gently over a low heat until the eggs are almost scrambled. Add the spinach and feta and continue to stir for another minute or so. (Try serving your eggs slightly moist and 'sloppy'. It doesn't sound very appetising but I think it tastes better.) Serve immediately in a bowl. No toast required. For a fresh taste, try sprinkling with chopped chives and parsley.

Variation

Add a handful of grated Cheddar cheese and some steamed broccoli florets instead of spinach and feta.

Homemade muesli

Makes one batch

Ingredients

- 1–2 handfuls porridge oats or spelt flakes
- 1–2 handfuls mixed nuts
- 1 handful mixed seeds (e.g. pumpkin and sunflower)
- 1 handful coconut flakes
- Optional extras: 1 tsp cinnamon, 2 tbsp raw cacao nibs or 2 tbsp chia seeds

Instructions

Mix all the ingredients together and store in an airtight container.

Foolproof smoothie

When blending smoothies, make leafy greens and vegetables the star of the show rather than fruit. Make sure you include some fat and protein too. Fat helps your body absorb the goodness from green vegetables, and fats and proteins make the smoothie more filling.

Work your way down the list below, choosing an item from each category, and you'll whizz up a perfect smoothie every time.

Ingredients

Liquid base (choose one)

- Coconut milk
- Almond milk
- Coconut water

Vegetable (choose one to three)

- A handful of spinach, watercress, rocket, kale or bok choy
- ½ cucumber
- 2–3 sticks of celery
- Small handful of parsley or mint

Fruit (choose one)

- 3 strawberries:
- 1 handful of frozen or fresh mixed berries
- ½ –1 apple
- ½ –1 banana
- 1 kiwi fruit
- 1 slice of pineapple
- 1 pear

Protein (choose one or two)

- 1 raw egg
- 1 tbsp full-fat plain yoghurt or Greek yoghurt
- 1 tbsp organic peanut butter or almond butter
- 1 tbsp nuts or seeds

Fat (choose one or two)

- 1 small ripe avocado
- 1–2 tbsp coconut (flakes or desiccated)
- 1–2 tbsp hemp oil or coconut oil

Optional extras (choose one or two)

- 1 tsp of chia seeds
- 2 tsp green powder such as spirulina
- ½ tsp ground cinnamon
- A pinch of vanilla powder or ¼ teaspoon of vanilla extract
- A pinch of stevia or a little honey
- 1–2 tbsp raw cacao powder
- Squeeze of lemon or lime
- 1 tsp fresh or ground ginger

If using root vegetables and apples, grating the vegetables first before blending will give a much smoother result. For a refreshing, cold smoothie, try using frozen banana or berries.

> *'I used to eat cereal but I've recently changed to a protein shake which I make with fruit, coconut milk, nuts, etc. With the old breakfast I'd be hungry by mid-morning and looking for a quick fix, which was typically none too healthy. My new breakfast keeps me going much longer – it's midday before I need anything else and having had a healthy start it's easier to continue with a healthy lunch.'*
>
> Mike

Breakfast for kids

Children might not be keen on giving up their high-sugar cereals, but their taste buds will soon adapt. Try weaning them off their usual cereals by switching to low-sugar cereals to begin with and then moving on to low-sugar alternatives such as homemade muesli, chopped fruit with nuts and yoghurt, and cooked breakfasts.

A great way to get kids on board is to get them involved:

- Ask them to help you make up jars of homemade muesli and let them choose which nuts and seeds to use.
- Take them shopping with you and ask them to become a Sugar Detective and find the 'good' sugar-free foods (yoghurt, cereal, etc.).
- Prepare as much as you can the night before and ask children to join in by getting the dishes and utensils ready on the breakfast table.
- Avoid stigmatising sugar and obsessing about it. Have fun to begin with but then let your sugar-free approach become the norm, rather than being something to shout about.

Chapter 11
Mid-morning Munchies

'At 11 a.m. I see what cakes they have at the coffee bar. It's so easy to get caught up in the "sugar fix" for a quick rush and then crash.'
Jason

'I crave pastries, chocolate, cheesecake, dried fruit – anything that I identify as a quick-fix pick-me-up.'
Katie

'I crave carbs and sugary stuff when I'm feeling depressed or bored at work.'
Rachel

'I have my "salad in a can". It's a tin of chickpeas, sweetcorn and tuna with a homemade oil-based salad dressing. It's nutritious and keeps me full until 2 p.m. It's an easy option so I never have the excuse to eat bad food between meetings.'
Mike

Soon after eating a high-sugar breakfast, we're likely to come down with the munchies. At this point, we're not interested in a gourmet three-course meal; we want something that's easy, instant and tasty. Enter chocolate bars, biscuits and sugary drinks. The energy from these snacks is short-lived. Once insulin kicks in, our blood-glucose levels crash, leaving us feeling tired and irritable, and craving yet another sugar fix. Muesli bars, dried fruit and flavoured yoghurts seem like the healthy option. But a glance at their food labels tells a very different story.

Are you on the sugar rollercoaster?

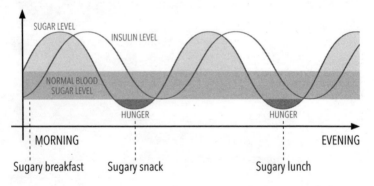

Sugar traps

Cereal bars

Many energy bars, cereal bars and fruit bars contain so much sugar they would be more at home in a sweet shop! A Nakd Rhubarb and Custard bar contains over 4 teaspoons of sugar. An Alpen Blueberry and Cranberry bar contains over 8 teaspoons.

Warning signs to look out for:

- Check the ingredients list. 'Sugar-free' bars usually contain fruit sugars from dried fruits like dates, which means they're packed full of fructose.

- If a bar doesn't contain fruit, it will be sweetened with *something* – honey, agave, maple syrup, cane sugar, artificial sweeteners.

Dried fruit

We looked at dried fruit in **Chapter 3**, but to quickly recap: dried fruit such as currants, dates, sultanas and figs are stripped of their water content, which concentrates the fruit sugars. Two 35 g fresh apricots contain around 1½ teaspoons of sugar, whereas 75 g of dried apricots contains over 7 teaspoons. Go for whole fruit over dried fruit every time.

Yoghurt

We've grown up thinking that fruit and yoghurt are good for us, so it stands to reason that we'd think fruit yoghurts are healthy. Here's the real deal on yoghurt:

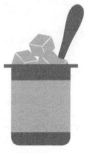

- A yoghurt with **'no added sugar'** emblazoned across its label may not contain cane sugar, but it will contain some form of 'fruit juice extract' or 'fruit juice concentrate' instead.

- Avoid **'diet' or 'low-fat'** yoghurts. When manufacturers take fat out of their product they put more sugar in to compensate for the lost flavour and texture. As a result, low-fat yogurts often contain more sugar than ice cream (along with dubious synthetic sweeteners).

- The solution? Eat plain, full-fat yoghurt or Greek yoghurt and add chopped fruit. Plain yoghurt should taste tart. If it's suspiciously sweet-tasting, check the ingredients list for signs of sugar being sneaked in in various guises.

The table below shows the sugar content of flavoured yoghurts. As a comparison, two scoops of Wall's Soft Scoop Vanilla Ice Cream contain just over 2 teaspoons of sugar.

High-sugar yoghurts

Yoghurt	Sugar content
Dannon Fruit on the Bottom – Blueberry	6 teaspoons per 170 g pot
Yeo Valley Organic Fat Free Yoghurt – Vanilla (450 g)	4½ teaspoons per 120 g serving
Tesco Finest B/Berry, Raspberry & Cranberry Yoghurt (400 g)	4½ teaspoons per 120 g serving
Müller Vitality Yoghurt – Strawberry	4 teaspoons per 120 g pot
Benecol Fat Free Garden Fruits Yoghurt	3 teaspoons per 120 g pot

Remember, some of the sugar listed above will be lactose (milk sugar). According to the National Dairy Council, the lactose content of yoghurt is generally *lower* than that of milk – which is 4.7 g of lactose per 100 g – so much of the sugar in flavoured yoghurts will be added sugar. Always check the ingredients list to be sure.

Low-sugar snacks

Snack enthusiasts argue that we should eat frequently throughout the day in order to stabilise our blood sugar levels. This used to be a virtually universally accepted rule, but it is now being challenged. New research shows that people who eat fewer, larger meals have lower blood glucose levels on average. They also tend to feel more satiated after eating compared with people who eat frequent meals and snacks. If you think about it, this makes sense – our ancient ancestors weren't able to pop down to the local supermarket whenever they felt like it. Our bodies have not evolved to constantly snack throughout the day.

Once you've been sugar-free for a few weeks, you should find your urge to snack nose-dives – providing you are eating a combination of good-quality proteins, fats and complex carbohydrates such as fruit and vegetables to fill you up. Listen to your body. If you're genuinely hungry, eat something, but stick to real (unprocessed) foods. Here are a few ideas to get you started:

Snack ideas

- Nuts
- 1–2 hard-boiled eggs
- Olives
- A piece of cheese
- Slice of smoked salmon
- Coconut flakes
- Homemade flapjack (see apple and coconut flapjack recipe later on in this chapter)

- Celery sticks dipped in nut butter
- Vegetables crudités with hummus (see recipe) or guacamole (see recipe)
- Leftover cold meat such as chicken drumsticks dipped in mustard
- Mini salad of mozzarella, tomatoes, basil leaves and olive oil
- Canned tuna or sardines with mashed avocado on sourdough toast

Mindfulness reminder

It's often our emotions that drive our snacking. There are two mindful eating techniques in **Chapter 9** that can really help – technique 1 (Eat when you're genuinely hungry) and 2 (Eat what your body needs). If you regularly practise tuning in to your body to see if your hunger is genuine, and then consult your gut and ask it what it needs, you'll find it easier to spot snacking that stems from emotional hunger and then be in a position to address this with something other than food.

Habit reminder

Snacking is often a habit we've fallen into. Experiment with some of the new habits below and you should feel the pull of your old habits start to weaken:

- **Habit 1:** Be prepared. Take healthy snacks to work with you or keep some in your bag if you're out for the day.

- **Habit 2:** Don't put snacks where you can see them – especially not lined up on your desk, waiting for you to munch your way through them!

- **Habit 3:** Don't put snacks within easy reach. Store them away from the kettle/tea-making area.

- **Habit 4:** Replace tins of biscuits or chocolate with a jar of mixed nuts and coconut flakes*.

- **Habit 5:** Avoid habit-inducing environments as much as possible. Unless you have Herculean willpower, avoid areas of the office where biscuits and birthday cakes are laid out to tempt you.

- **Habit 6:** Avoid habit-inducing behaviours. Instead of catching up with friends over tea and cake, offer to meet for a walk instead.

- **Habit 7:** Distract yourself. Go for a walk round the block, drink some water, hang out the washing, phone a friend, ask a friend or loved one for a hug.

*Nuts and coconut are both nutrient-rich foods. You don't need to eat much to quell any hunger pangs. As with any food, if you binge on them, you may put on weight. Stick to one small handful a day.

Exercise reminder

A mid-morning break is the perfect time to fit in a 10-minute burst of exercise: go for a quick walk outside or walk up and down some stairs. Move as much as you can throughout the day, e.g. walking the dog, gardening, housework, walking to the shops, stretching, playing golf. A 2010 analysis of ten different studies showed just 5 minutes of exercise is enough to have a mood-boosting effect. If you can head outdoors, even better – 5 minutes of 'green exercise' decreases stress, boosts mood, and enhances self-esteem!

Snacking for kids

Childhood is a time of rapid growth, and snacking plays an important part in meeting a child's nutritional needs. Here are some ideas for fun, healthy snacks:

- **Ants on a log:** Spread nut butter on half a stick of celery and dot nuts or olives over the butter.

- **Ladybirds on a log:** As above but use chopped strawberries instead of nuts/olives.

- **Fruit and cheese stars:** Use a small star-shaped cookie cutter to cut stars from slices of cheese and fruit (e.g. melon and apple).

- **Orange and green chips:** Roast sweet potato chips and serve with a green dip (mashed avocado with a squeeze of lemon or lime juice).

- **Apple teeth:** Spread two slices of apple ('lips') with nut butter and stick chopped banana ('teeth') between the slices.

- **Hedgehog hummus:** Stick lots of thin batons of carrots, celery and pepper in a pot of hummus (add two raw cacao nibs or black olives for eyes if you're feeling extra creative!).

Snack recipes

Hummus

Makes one batch

Ingredients

- 1 x 400 g tin of chickpeas, drained
- 1 garlic clove, crushed or finely chopped
- Juice of ½ a lemon
- 2 tbsp of extra virgin olive oil
- 1 tbsp of sesame seeds
- Sea salt and black pepper

Instructions

Blend all the ingredients together and add lemon juice and seasoning to taste. Add some water or a little more oil if the consistency is too thick.

Guacamole

Makes one batch

Ingredients

- 2 large, ripe avocados
- 1 garlic clove, crushed or finely chopped
- 1 tbsp of extra virgin olive oil
- Juice of 1 lime
- Sea salt and black pepper
- Optional: finely chopped green chilli, tomato, red onion and coriander

Instructions

Either blend all the ingredients together or, for a more chunky texture, mash the ingredients in a bowl. Add lemon juice, oil and seasoning to taste.

Apple and coconut flapjacks*

Serves 8–10

Ingredients

- 140 g rolled oats
- 50 g desiccated coconut
- 2 apples (seeds removed, unpeeled, chopped into quarters)
- 2 tbsp chopped nuts (e.g. pecans or walnuts)
- 1 tbsp honey (or sweetener of your choice)
- 2 tbsp coconut oil
- 1–2 tsp ground cinnamon (optional)

Instructions

Puree the apples in a food processor with a tablespoon of water. Melt the coconut oil and honey in a saucepan, remove from the heat and add the pureed apples and remaining ingredients and mix well. Grease a cake tin with a little coconut oil and press the mixture into the tin. Bake in the oven at 180°C for around 20 minutes or until golden. Leave to cool, then cut into slices.

*Note: These flapjacks do contain honey (a very small amount per slice) but they are far more nutritious than chocolate bars and most commercial cereal bars.

Chapter 12
Lunch

'My worst habit is wanting to eat something sweet after meals, particularly after lunch at work or when I am tired while driving long distances.'
Denyse

'Planning my meals helps – not leaving it to the work canteen where healthy eating is very difficult.'
Katie

'I crave cheesy puffs! If I'm feeling stressed about a big job, this is what I want in the bowl on my desk.'
Eileen

Lunchtime used to be a leisurely affair, but nowadays the lunch break is practically extinct. Just one in five of us takes an hour-long lunch break, and 60 per cent of us opt to eat at our desks. No wonder our favourite lunchtime food is the humble sandwich; one of the easiest handheld, portable foods.

In the UK, we buy 3 billion ready-made sandwiches a year! After selecting our favourite filling (chicken, closely followed by ham and egg, according to surveys), how many of us think to stop and scrutinise the list of ingredients for sugar? Sandwiches and sugar just don't seem to go together. It's a similar story for soups, salads and flavoured water. As is often the case with sugar, all is not what it seems.

Sugar traps

Sandwiches

We feel safe with a sandwich – bread, salad, meat, cheese… what could go wrong? Well, an innocent little cheese and chutney sandwich can contain 5 teaspoons of sugar. There's also the fact that bread (wraps, baguettes, paninis, bagels, ciabattas and rolls) is quickly converted into glucose in the body, so it raises blood sugar levels. It sounds like there's no escape, but you can offset some of this by choosing the right types of bread and fillings.

Healthy sandwiches

- Stick to low-sugar breads such as sourdough or rye, or wholemeal pitta if possible.

- Omit the bread altogether and serve the sandwich filling on little gem lettuce leaves, or buy high-protein sushi if you're out and about.

- Choose protein fillings – such as meat, tuna, egg or prawn – which balance out the meal and slow down the release of sugar.

- Watch out for dressings and sauces – especially pickles, chutneys, sweet chilli and hoisin sauce.

When making sandwiches at home…

- Get out of a sandwich rut by trying different ingredients – spinach, watercress or rocket, with shredded carrots, black olives, hummus and sliced avocado for example.
- Use low- or no-sugar spreads such as mustard, olive oil, butter, nut butter, tapenade, hummus, guacamole, Marmite or organic peanut butter.

Crisps

Figures from market research company Mintel reveal that we eat a tonne of crisps every 3 minutes in the UK (enough to fill a telephone box every 43 seconds). This might have something to do with the fact that crisps are designed to be addictive. Manufacturers make sure their crisps have just the right combination of salt, fat and sugar that our brain craves. There's also the scientifically honed crispiness. Research has found that the more noise a crisp makes when you bite into it, the more you will like it. So manufacturers make sure their crisps have the perfect crave-inducing crunch (we love crisps that snap with 4 pounds of pressure per square inch, if you're interested).

But hang on, what have crisps got to do with sugar? Fat and salt might be a concern when buying crisps, but sugar is usually the last thing on our mind. Most crisps are made from potato… and potatoes are a starchy carbohydrate… and carbohydrates get broken down into glucose in the body… and, well, you know the rest. Whether crisps are 'natural' or not, and whether they are baked or fried, they will *all* influence your insulin levels in a very negative way. Add tooth decay and weight gain into the mix, and crisps don't look quite so appealing – crisps can stick to the surface of teeth for hours, and in America, crisps are being cited as one of the largest contributors to the obesity epidemic.

Healthier crisps:

- If you eat shop-bought crisps, eat them rarely (not every day).
- Crisps with the strongest flavours tend to be the highest in sugar.
- Steer clear of obviously sweet flavours, such as sweet chilli.
- Always read the ingredients list before you buy and remember, even if the sugar content appears to be low, carbohydrates such as potatoes, rice, corn (tortillas) and wheat (pretzels) break down into sugars.
- Better yet, make your own crisps – then you can guarantee the ingredients (see recipes below).

Alternatives to crisps and how to make them at home

Kale chips

Makes one portion

Ingredients

- 2 large handfuls kale
- 1 tbsp olive oil or coconut oil
- Sea salt to taste

Instructions

Remove any tough stalks from the kale and tear into rough pieces. Mix with 1 tablespoon of olive oil and sea salt to taste. Arrange in a single layer on a baking sheet, and roast until crisp (around 10 minutes). Sprinkle with a little sea salt and eat immediately.

Sweet potato crisps

Makes one portion

Ingredients

- 1–2 sweet potatoes
- 1 tsp coconut oil
- Seasoning to taste (sea salt, chilli powder/flakes or cumin)

Instructions

Thinly slice a sweet potato (keeping the skin on) using a potato peeler or mandolin. Oil a baking tray with coconut oil and cook at 200°C for 10 minutes turning halfway through. Season with sea salt, chilli powder or flakes, or cumin. Try roasting with sliced parsnips and beetroot for mixed vegetable crisps.

Curried almonds

Makes one portion

Ingredients

- 2 handfuls almonds
- 1 tsp turmeric
- ½ tsp ground cumin
- ½ tsp ground coriander
- Black pepper and sea salt

Instructions

Heat 2 handfuls of almonds in 1 teaspoon of coconut oil. Stir in a good pinch of sea salt, 1 teaspoon of turmeric and ½ a teaspoon each of ground cumin and coriander. Toast gently for about 3 minutes until the spices are fragrant. Finish with a grind of black pepper. Remove from heat and allow to cool.

Fizzy and soft drinks

If you've opted for a lunchtime meal deal, your sandwich and crisps might be washed down with a fizzy drink. Research by Action on Sugar has found that nearly four out of five 330 ml servings of carbonated sugar-sweetened drinks contain more than 6 teaspoons of sugar. Seemingly healthier options such as flavoured water, elderflower, and traditional drinks such as ginger beer and cloudy lemonade, contain more sugar than Coca-Cola and Pepsi. Here are some examples:

Fizzy drink	Sugar content per 330 ml serving (equivalent to one can)
Jammin Sparkling Ginger Beer	12 teaspoons
Waitrose Cloudy Lemonade	10 teaspoons
Tesco Finest Grape & Elderflower Spritz	9 teaspoons
Coca-Cola	8 teaspoons
Amé Grape & Apricot	5 teaspoons
Volvic Juiced Berry Medley	5 teaspoons

Tips for drinking fizzy drinks:

- *Don't drink them!* I know that sounds harsh but they contain nothing of any nutritional value and they are one of THE worst things you can consume for your health. You would never pour yourself a glass of water and then add 6–12 teaspoons of sugar. But that's exactly what fizzy drink manufacturers do to every can.

- Maybe think about it like this: when we drink a fizzy drink, it's because we're thirsty and yet these drinks contain lots of calories. A can of standard cola contains between 140 and 150 calories. Some energy drinks can contain up to 200 calories per can. The average glass of water contains *zero* calories.
- Drink water instead.

Ways to make water more exciting

Try adding one or two of the following:

- A non-fruit* herbal teabag such as ginger or chamomile (let it steep in the cold water)
- Slices of apple and half a cinnamon stick
- Fresh basil and Angostura bitters
- Slices of fresh ginger, cucumber and celery
- Lemon, lime, grapefruit or orange slices
- Sparkling water with crushed raspberries and bruised mint leaves
- Sparkling water with strawberries, cucumber and mint

*Citric juice and fruit teas can be acidic to teeth if drunk frequently or in large amounts.

Salad dressings

Salads can be a nutritious option for lunch but some salad dressings are not quite as saintly as they seem. Many contain more than 12 per cent sugar, which means that a 30 ml serving (2 tablespoons) can dump a teaspoon of sugar unceremoniously onto your lunch.

Commercial salad dressings	Typical percentage sugar
Balsamic vinegar	20–40+ per cent
Balsamic vinaigrette	14–18 per cent
French	8–12 per cent
Thousand Island	11 per cent
Italian	8 per cent
Caesar	1–4 per cent
'Light' mayonnaise	2 per cent
Mayonnaise	1.5 per cent

Healthy salad dressings

There's no need to shun salad dressings altogether – they taste good and the fats help your body to absorb the antioxidants in vegetables (yet another reason to steer clear of 'low-fat' products). Just switch to some better oil-based alternatives to help you get the most nutritional value out of your meal, or make your own salad dressing in seconds:

- Use extra virgin olive oil or hemp oil as your base oil and add flavours (see below).

- Replace balsamic vinegar (high sugar) with unpasteurised apple cider vinegar, or red or white wine vinegar.

- Add garlic, herbs, mustard (wholegrain, French, Dijon), yoghurt, and/ or a squeeze of lemon, lime or orange juice, a pinch of sea salt and black pepper.

Soups and baked beans

Soups can be a healthy option, especially if you make them yourself. Watch out for shop-bought versions, particularly tomato-based soups and tomato-based sauces in tins of baked beans and spaghetti. Tomatoes contain natural sugar but if slightly unripe tomatoes are used in soups and sauces, they can have an acidic taste. Sugar is added to soften this.

Soup	Sugar content
Cream of tomato soup	2½ teaspoons (half a 400 g can)
Tomato and basil soup	4 teaspoons per serving (half a 600 g carton)
Baked beans	2½–3 teaspoons per serving (half a 400 g can)
Spaghetti in tomato sauce	2 teaspoons per serving (half a 400 g can)

Tips for healthy soups:

- Avoid canned products as they have sugar added to extend their shelf life.
- Watch out for artificial sweeteners in low-sugar soups.
- Ideally, cook your own vegetable soup at home and freeze it in separate portions, ready for lunch during the week. Add meat, chickpeas or lentils to turn it into a more filling stew.

Low- or no-sugar lunches

There's no doubt that making your own lunch requires more planning than rushing to the shops and grabbing the nearest thing that jumps off the shelf. But making your own lunch puts you back in control. And it needn't be complicated. It could be as simple as preparing a salad the night before and putting it in the fridge ready to take to work the next day (see recipes at the end of this chapter).

Lunch ideas

Salad

Generous salads using a variety of salad leaves, roasted vegetables, protein (fish, meat, cheese, nuts, seeds, boiled eggs) and a dressing (see recipes at the end of this chapter).

Soup

Vegetable soup with added protein (i.e. meat, fish, chickpeas, grated parmesan topping).

Sandwich

- Leftover roasted vegetables, spinach, guacamole and feta or goat's cheese
- Roasted butternut squash, onion, chicken, spinach, harissa-spiked sugar-free mayo
- Hummus, grated carrot, pine nuts, coriander and rocket

Egg

- Vegetable frittata and salad
- Any of the 'cooked breakfast' suggestions plus a side salad

Fish

- Mackerel or sardine pâté on sourdough toast with watercress (see recipe at the end of this chapter)
- Mackerel or trout fillet with walnuts, salad, homemade mustard mayonnaise and avocado
- Smoked salmon, crab, sardines or tuna mixed with homemade coleslaw served on little gem lettuce leaves

Meat

- Two cold chicken drumsticks with mustard, served with vegetable crudités and hummus
- Homemade coleslaw with salad and any meat or fish

Sushi

Jacket potato or sweet potato (topped with protein*)

- Hummus and parsley
- Chicken and homemade coleslaw
- Flaked mackerel and lemon crème fraiche

*Both sweet potatoes and jacket potatoes are high in carbohydrate but you can make the meal more balanced by eating the skin, adding a protein and/ or fat topping, and eating smaller potatoes and larger fillings, perhaps with a side salad.

Mindfulness reminder

There can be so many distractions at lunchtime. We're often eating on the run, working at our desks, or immersed in our own mental chatter. Mindful eating technique 4 (Focus on your food) will multiply the pleasure you get from eating your lunch and will help you to feel more satisfied. Try it and you'll be surprised how it leaves you feeling calm and focused, ready for the afternoon.

Habits reminder

- Plan your lunches and add the ingredients you need to your weekly shopping list – if you have all the ingredients to hand, you'll be less likely to throw a wobbly and succumb to convenience food.

- Make as much as possible the night before (e.g. a salad to which you add a dressing and nuts the next morning before you head off to work).

- Freeze soups and stews in individual portions and take out at night to defrost ready for the next day.

Exercise reminder

British researcher Jim McKenna from Leeds Metropolitan University has found that when people exercise in their lunch hour they are less likely to experience a 'post-lunch dip' (added bonus: their performance at work also improves by 15 per cent). It doesn't seem to matter what sort of exercise you do. In Jim's study of 210 office workers in England, participants did 45–60 minutes of an activity of their choice, including stretching, yoga, aerobics, strength training and basketball. 'It's the paradox of exercise,' he says, 'to get energy you have to expend some.'

Lunch for kids

A survey by consumer watchdog Which? found that the food in a child's lunchbox can contain as much sugar as ten McDonald's sugar doughnuts! A packed lunch made up of five seemingly healthy items, including cheese and biscuits and fruit juice, contained 12 teaspoons of sugar. Here are some naturally sweet alternatives:

- Sweet potato crisps (sliced and baked in the oven)
- Baby carrots and sweet red pepper hummus dip
- Raw sweet vegetables such as cherry tomatoes, sugar snap peas, corn on the cob
- Apple and coconut flapjack (see recipe in **Chapter 11**)
- Apple slices dipped in macadamia or cashew nut butter
- Homemade banana bread or blueberry muffin.

Recipes

As with smoothies, there's a foolproof way to build a satisfying salad:

1. Use a variety of **salad leaves** (chicory, watercress, baby spinach, rocket).

2. Add some **protein** (fish, seafood, meat, cheese, nuts, seeds, boiled eggs).

3. Add some **fat** (avocado, olives, nuts, seeds, extra virgin olive oil or hemp oil).

4. Add dense **vegetables** such as peppers, cauliflower, broccoli and spring onions or leftover roasted vegetables.

Chicory and parmesan salad

Serves 2

Ingredients

- 1 chicory, chopped into large pieces
- Handful of cress or watercress
- 2 celery sticks, sliced
- Handful of sugar snap peas, chopped in half
- Handful of frozen peas (cooked and then cooled in cold water)

Topping

- Small handful of nuts (e.g. pine nuts and chopped walnuts)
- Small handful of pumpkin seeds
- Small handful of parmesan or pecorino shavings (or chopped feta or goat's cheese)
- 2 tbsp homemade dressing

Instructions

Mix the ingredients together and sprinkle the topping ingredients over the top.

Grated salad

Serves 2

Ingredients

- 2 carrots, grated
- 1 courgette, grated
- 1 spring onion, chopped
- A few cauliflower florets, chopped
- Handful of cherry tomatoes
- Small handful of pumpkin seeds
- Small handful of sunflower seeds
- Small handful of chopped walnuts
- 2 tbsp homemade dressing
- Plus one or two of the following: a boiled egg, a tin of tuna, some cheese, nuts, or half an avocado

Instructions

Mix all the ingredients together in bowl and serve.

Homemade salad dressing

Makes 180 ml (around half a jam jar)

Ingredients

- 60 ml apple cider vinegar
- 120 ml extra virgin olive oil
- Pinch of salt and pepper
- ½ clove of garlic, crushed
- Pinch of dried herbs such as oregano, marjoram or tarragon
- Chopped fresh herbs such as parsley, mint, chives or basil

Optional extra flavours

- Choose one or two of the following:
- 1 tsp Dijon mustard
- ½ tsp honey/brown rice syrup

Instructions

Pour the above ingredients into a clean jam jar, shake well and store in the fridge for up to a week.

Mackerel pâté and watercress on toast

Serves 2–3

Ingredients

- 3 smoked mackerel fillets
- 3 tbsp plain or Greek yoghurt
- Juice of ½ a lemon
- 1 tbsp capers
- Black pepper
- Watercress
- Cayenne pepper (optional)

Instructions

Remove the skin from three smoked mackerel fillets and flake them into a blender or a bowl with 3 tbsp of plain or Greek yoghurt, the juice of ½ a lemon, 1 tablespoon of chopped capers, and a grind of black pepper. Blend to form a rough texture (or mash in a bowl with a fork). Toast some sourdough or rye bread, top with watercress and then the mackerel pâté. Finish with a sprinkling of cayenne pepper. To add extra spice, try adding a little bit of Tabasco sauce or horseradish to the mix.

Chapter 13
Afternoon Slump

> 'I've stopped drinking Diet Coke in the afternoon.
> Although technically it contains no sugar, it sends
> the cravings through the roof!'
>
> Katie

> 'Sometimes I have a craving for a "sugar hit"
> but it doesn't really matter what it is as long as it has
> sugar in it. I have even been known to have a spoonful
> of toffee ice cream sauce in desperate times!'
>
> George

If you find yourself running out of steam halfway through the afternoon, it could be due to a number of things. It could be that you ate lots of sugary food earlier in the day and are on the sugar roller coaster, hurtling downwards towards a dip. It could be the fact that you didn't sleep well the previous night and your appetite control mechanisms are out of whack. Or it could be due to your body temperature and cortisol levels dipping between 2 p.m. and 4 p.m. as part of your body's 24-hour cycle or circadian rhythm. Regardless of the cause, there's one end result: by mid-afternoon we feel tired and sluggish, and a sugary cup of tea with biscuits seems like a remarkably good idea. But this is the opposite of what our body needs. Sugary snacks give us a short burst of energy – and before we know it we're heading for another energy slump.

Sugar traps

Hot drinks

One of the problems with buying sweet drinks from a café or canteen is that you'll have very little idea of what's actually in them – unless, that is, you happen to buy your drink from a high-street chain that posts its nutritional data on its website. Here are some examples from Starbucks and Costa (all made with skimmed milk):

Drink	Sugar content (grams)	Sugar content (teaspoons)*
Costa (450 ml 'Medio')		
Café latte	15.6 g	4
Mocha	35 g	8
Hot chocolate	35.7 g	8½
Cinnamon latte	27 g	6½
Starbucks (470 ml, 'Grande')		
Caramel macchiato	31.9 g	7½

White chocolate mocha with whipped cream	59.9 g	14
Chai tea latte	42 g	10
Cappuccino	10.3 g	2½

*Note: Sugar content (teaspoons) figures are rounded to the nearest half.

Try these tips to reduce your sugar intake:

- Either go cold turkey and resolutely refuse to add any sugar to your tea or coffee, or take the small-steps approach and gradually reduce the amount you add each day in order to give your taste buds time to adjust.

- If you buy your hot drinks in a high-street coffee shop, take a look at the nutritional information listed on their website and switch to a low-sugar drink, e.g. replace your white chocolate mocha with a standard mocha – obviously, this doesn't mean the drink is good for you; just that you're reducing your sugar intake!

- As you would expect, the best options to go for are the plainest teas and coffees (fresh filtered coffee, Americano and espresso).

- Try sprinkling cinnamon on your cappuccino instead of sugar. Cinnamon helps stabilise blood sugar levels and adds flavour without the sweetness.

- Swap sugary hot drinks for sweet-tasting herbal teas such as chai, vanilla, cinnamon and cardamom.

Biscuits, cakes and chocolate bars

Coffee and a biscuit, tea and a slice of cake – hot drinks often trigger some of our worst sugar habits. This is how much sugar is lurking in some of our most popular cakes, biscuits and chocolate bars:

Product	Sugar per serving
Carrot cake	5–7 teaspoons per slice
Chocolate cake	5–7 teaspoons per slice
McVitie's Milk Chocolate Digestives biscuit	1 teaspoon per biscuit
Jacob's Club Mint biscuit	2 teaspoons per biscuit
Dairy Milk chocolate bar	6 teaspoons per bar (45 g)
Snickers chocolate bar	6½ teaspoons per bar (53 g)

Biscuit guidelines:

- Beware of 'low-fat' or 'diet' biscuits. Biscuits with reduced fat taste like cardboard, so manufacturers up the sugar content to add flavour.

- To reduce your sugar intake, you could switch to a savoury biscuit such as oatcakes or multigrain crackers topped with plain butter, salmon, tuna, cheese or nut butter. (Remember the insulin response; these are carbohydrates).

- The healthiest option is to ditch the biscuits, cakes and bars and make your own homemade bars (see **Chapter 11** for more snack ideas and an apple and coconut flapjack recipe).

Mindfulness reminder

A snack can be gone within a few mindless bites. However, a snack's small size means it's the perfect focus for a burst of high-intensity attention. By focusing 100 per cent on the sight, smell, texture, taste and sound of your food or drink as you bite or sip, you can derive maximum pleasure from your snack (which should mean less of an urge for a second helping). Look back at the 'Mini food or drink meditation' in **Chapter 9** for further instructions.

Habit reminder

The following healthy habits will help you ward off a mid-afternoon slump:

- **Get a good night's sleep**. It's thought that our body rejuvenates between the hours of 11 p.m. and 1 a.m. (particularly our adrenal glands which release hormones in response to stress), so aim to be asleep by 11 p.m.

- **Include protein-rich foods and healthy fats** in your breakfast and lunch. This will help to fill you up and keep you going through the afternoon.

- **Get outside** at lunchtime and stretch your legs – the movement and exposure to natural light will refresh you for the afternoon.

- **Keep your fluid levels topped up**. Dehydration causes drowsiness. Don't wait until you're thirsty to have a drink because by then you are already dehydrated.

- **Get up and move**. If you work in an office, at least once an hour, get up from your desk. Schedule physical chores for the afternoon – you could walk to the post office or shops, for example.

- **Consider a stand-up work desk**. This needn't be an elaborate or expensive affair – at home I put my laptop on the kitchen sideboard on top of the polystyrene box that housed my new printer.

- **Stretch**. Stretching limbs stimulates the brain and reinvigorates us.

Exercise reminder

Did you know that after just 90 minutes of sitting your metabolism shuts down? Or that if you sit for 8 hours a day your risk of contracting heart disease, cancer and diabetes rises by 40 per cent? This is due to the fact that sitting for several hours at a time lowers your metabolic rate, reduces sensitivity to insulin, and shuts down your fat-burning system. But the good news is there is something incredibly simple you can do to counteract the negative effects of sitting down all day – **stand up every 15 minutes!** It may seem insignificant, but standing up requires big changes in your body – your muscles contract, your bones are stimulated and your heart rate increases. Even raising your arms above your head and stretching will help.

Low- or no-sugar snack ideas

As usual, listen to your body. If you're genuinely hungry and really need a snack, stick to real rather than processed food – see 'Snack ideas' in **Chapter 11**.

Snacking for kids

Experts recommend avoiding using sweets as a reward for good behaviour or as a way to calm an upset child. This can lead to an unhealthy emotional connection between eating certain foods and feeling good. Instead of rewarding kids with food, reward them with a fun activity:

- A trip to the swings or play centre
- Playing a favourite game
- A swim in the local pool
- New art supplies or colouring book
- Going to the beach
- Reading a favourite story together
- Doing some cooking
- A trip to the library
- A play date or sleepover with a friend

Chapter 14
Dinner

'My worst habit is eating cakes and biscuits when I'm really, really tired instead of going to bed early at night.'
Karen

'I crave sugar/chocolate late at night or when I'm tired at the end of the day.'
Joe

'I find it difficult to find alternative sweet puddings!'
Anna

'I have cheese curls and wine in the evening as justification for having had a very boring day at work.'
Derek

> *'I crave carbs when I'm tired and chocolate after I've eaten dinner.'*
> Karen

Have you ever come home at the end of the day and felt so tired (or stressed) it felt like a monumental effort just to decide what to eat for supper, let alone physically prepare anything? According to NHS figures, one in five of us say we feel tired all the time. It's such a common complaint, doctors use an acronym on their patient notes: TATT. Exhaustion combined with work pressures and family commitments make takeaways and ready-made meals a tempting option, but many contain high levels of sugar and have dubious nutritional content! (That's me being diplomatic. A recent study by the *British Medical Journal* analysed 100 supermarket own-brand ready meals and found that none of them complied with nutritional guidelines set by the World Health Organization.)

Reducing our sugar intake and keeping our blood sugar levels on an even keel can make a massive difference to our energy levels, but we're often too tired to cook meals from scratch, so we get caught in a vicious cycle.

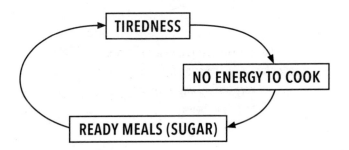

Sugar traps

Takeaways

Guess what the nation's favourite takeaway is? Surprisingly, it's not Indian; it's Chinese. Indian comes in second place, followed by fish and chips and then pizza. Our two favourite takeaways happen to be the ones most loaded with sugar. The average chicken tikka masala contains 8 teaspoons of sugar and a Cantonese sweet and sour chicken contains an incredible 16 teaspoons. That's not including any sugar in the fried rice. And let's not mention the fat, salt and food-colouring content.

Healthier takeaways:

- When Which? tested the sugar content of Chinese, Indian and pizza takeaways, it found Chinese takeaways contained nearly three times as much sugar as an Indian meal. Pizza contained the least sugar by far.

- It's not all good news for pizza, though. Most pizzas contain processed flour in the base which can cause blood sugar to rise rapidly. Stick to thin-crust pizzas.

- Steer clear of obviously sweet meals such as kormas and peshwari naans, and sweet and sour or sweet chilli sauces. Low-sugar dishes include dry curries such as tandoori with plain naan, and Chinese soups with steamed vegetables and prawns.

- Remember, some of the sugar in products may be naturally occurring in fruit, such as the pineapple used in sweet and sour chicken and pizzas, so take this into consideration when choosing between different products.

- The healthiest option of all is of course to reserve takeaways for rare occasions and switch to home-cooked food. You don't need to be slaving away for hours. Check out the recipe books listed in the **Resources** chapter at the end of this book or try the quick pizza ideas below (great for kids too).

Cheat's tomato sauce

Ingredients

- Can of chopped tomatoes
- 1 tsp of coconut oil
- 1 clove of garlic, sliced
- Handful of fresh basil
- Salt and pepper to season

Instructions

Gently fry the sliced garlic in a little coconut oil for 1–2 minutes. Add a can of chopped tomatoes, a handful of torn basil leaves (or dried basil) and simmer gently until the sauce has reduced. Add sea salt and pepper and serve. You can make this in big batches and freeze it in portions.

Mini pizzas

Serves 1

Ingredients

- 2 tbsp tomato puree (or home-made tomato sauce)
- 2 wholemeal pittas
- A few spinach leaves, wilted
- A few fresh mint leaves, torn
- A few black olives
- Handful of cherry tomatoes
- Some chopped red pepper and/or red onion
- Some feta cheese, crumbled
- ½–1 clove of garlic, chopped
- Salt and pepper to season

Instructions

Smear the tomato puree or homemade tomato sauce on a wholemeal pitta and add 2–3 torn mint leaves and a few leaves of wilted spinach. Top with black olives, chopped garlic, cherry tomatoes and crumbled feta. Season with salt and pepper and pop under the grill for 5 minutes or so until the cheese is lightly toasted.

Cauliflower pizza base

Serves 2

Ingredients

- 1 medium cauliflower
- 1 egg
- 100 g goat's cheese or grated Cheddar
- Salt and pepper to season

Instructions

Grate a medium-sized cauliflower, cook in boiling water for a few minutes, drain well and mix with 1 egg, 100 g of goat's cheese or grated Cheddar cheese and some salt and pepper. Shape the mixture into bases (roughly 1 cm thick), place on baking paper and bake for 30 minutes in the oven until golden and firm. Add your favourite topping and bake for 8–10 minutes. You can also use baked portobello mushrooms or sliced aubergines for your base, as an alternative.

Ready-meals and jars of sauce

Analysis by Which? reveals that many supermarket ready meals contain up to 10 teaspoons of sugar. A small 45 g bar of milk chocolate contains a mere 6 teaspoons of sugar in comparison. As you would expect, sweet and sour and sweet chilli meals are the worst offenders. Sweet and sour chicken with rice contains up to 12 teaspoons of sugar and chicken pad Thai with rice noodles contains up to 9 teaspoons. Many shop-bought sauces also contain added sugar. Here are a few examples:

Sauce	Sugar content (per 125 g)
Barbecue sauce	3 teaspoons
Tomato and herb pasta sauce	2 teaspoons
Green Thai curry sauce	1 teaspoon
Caribbean curry sauce	1 teaspoon
Creamy mushroom sauce	½ teaspoon

Healthier ready-made meals and sauces

- Always check the food label – buy products with no added sugar or sugar which appears very low down in the list of ingredients.

- If the list contains a long list of ingredients you can't pronounce, leave it on the shelf!

- Be aware that many ready meals contain two or more servings or portions. If you eat the whole pack, you'll need to multiply the sugar 'per serving' figure to calculate your sugar intake.

- Similarly, with jars of sauce, the figures in the above table may not seem too bad at first glance, but bear in mind that most of us don't use a 125 g serving of sauce; we use two–three times this amount.

Try this

To up your veggie intake and reduce wheat in your diet, try serving Bolognese and pasta sauces on strips of raw courgette rather than spaghetti or pasta shapes. Chop the ends of a courgette and use a peeler to slice thin strips (leave the skin on).

Desserts

It's clear we love our puddings – four in ten people in Britain go as far as to say that eating a pudding is better than sex! When we eat sugar the brain releases dopamine, a feel-good neurotransmitter. But what the brain really goes crazy for is a combination of fat *and* sugar (think chocolate bars and ice cream). Preliminary research reveals that high-sugar and high-fat foods work like heroin, opium and morphine in the brain, overwhelming our ordinary biological signals that control hunger. That's why the nation's favourite dessert isn't fruit salad; it's apple crumble, cheesecake and chocolate cake.

Healthier desserts

- At home, serve desserts in smaller bowls – this makes the portion look larger and can help fool the brain into thinking you've eaten more than you have.

- Switch to fresh desserts based on fruit and yoghurt. For example, a handful of chopped fruit topped with yoghurt, coconut flakes, toasted walnuts and a sprinkle of cinnamon.

- In restaurants, swap dessert for coffee or a cheese platter, or go for a starter and a main rather than a main and a dessert.

- Try drinking a sweet-tasting herbal tea to quell any urges for something sweet to eat (see suggestions in **Chapter 5**).

Alcohol

Everyone has an Achilles heel when it comes to their diet. If, like me, your Achilles heel is a glass of wine, you'll be relieved to discover that alcohol need not be banished altogether. You may simply want to tweak your drinking habits to ensure you're sipping less sugar.

A survey of drinks conducted in 2014 for the *Daily Telegraph* found a certain well-known Irish cream liqueur contained the highest concentration of sugar (5 teaspoons per 100 ml), followed by sherry and cider. In contrast, most of the wines, beers and champagnes analysed contained less than a teaspoon of sugar per glass.

In terms of sugar content, wine, beer and spirits are good choices as most of the natural sugars in fruits, grains and berries are converted to alcohol during the fermentation and distillation process. Dry cider is better than sweet, but it does contain more sugar than wine, beer or spirits.

Bad choices	Good choices
Dessert wines	Wine (especially dry)
Sherry	Beers and stouts
Port	Spirits (gin, vodka, whisky)
Sweet cider	Dry cider
Fruit cocktails	
Sweet liqueurs	
Mixers such as tonic water	

Tips for low-sugar drinks

- The drier the wine or cider the better.

- Red wine tends to retain less fructose than white.

- Beers and stouts contain maltose, not fructose, which is fine for us to digest (though some lagers and ales have added sugar or honey for additional flavouring so always check the nutritional information on the bottle).

- Champagne isn't a great option as it tends to retain more fructose.

- When drinking sparkling wine and champagne, go for extra dry, brut, or extra brut (extra brut is the driest).

- Beware of mixers such as tonic water and fruit juice, which can contain 8–10 teaspoons of sugar in one tall glass. Drink your spirits neat (in small quantities!) or mix with soda water instead.

- Avoid flavoured drinks such as ciders flavoured with cherry or raspberry.

Healthy drinking

Alcohol is high in empty calories and overuse is linked to a myriad of health issues, including metabolic syndrome, which affects an estimated one in four adults in the UK. (Metabolic syndrome is the medical term for a combination of diabetes, high blood pressure and obesity.) As you consume less sugar, you may find your tolerance for alcohol is lower. In the meantime, follow these guidelines:

- Don't drink on an empty stomach; drink with meals in order to slow down the rush of sugars to your liver.

- Stick to government safe-drinking guidelines: 3–4 units per day for a man (equivalent to a pint and a half of 4 per cent beer) and 2–3 units per day for a woman (equivalent to a 175 ml glass of 13 per cent wine).

- Have at least two alcohol-free days a week.

Low- or no-sugar supper ideas

The ideas below all make speedy weekday evening meals. One-pot dishes such as curries, pies and stews are perfect for saving washing-up and great for making in bulk and then freezing.

Dinner ideas

- Pork or lamb chop with stir-fried garlicky spring greens
- Marinated chicken breast (lemon and pepper) served with sweet potato chips and kale

- White fish fillet baked with green pesto and sliced lemon, served with steamed green veg
- Salmon fillet topped with red pesto, cherry tomatoes and black olives, served with green beans
- Vegetable or meat curry
- Vegetable stew
- Fish pie
- One-pot seafood or fish stew
- Homemade pizza
- Chinese stir-fry or broth
- Thai curry (add sugar free Thai green curry paste to coconut milk and cook with sliced red pepper, courgette, baby sweetcorn, chestnut mushrooms, green beans, lime and coriander)
- Baked sweet potato topped with hummus and parsley, served with a salad

Mindfulness reminder

Evening meals are often eaten on autopilot while watching TV or chatting. To tap into your body's hunger signals, try technique number six from **Chapter 9**; 'Eat until you are satiated (not stuffed)'. When nearing the end of a meal, focus on your stomach and gauge how full you feel on a scale of one to ten. Stop eating when you reach seven or imagine your stomach as being 70–80 per cent full.

Habits reminder

Did you know that if you wake often during the night or wake up tired it could be due to the chocolate you ate after dinner? Snacking on sugars and grains before bed raises blood sugar levels, and at some point during the night they will come crashing back down again. It's a repeat of your afternoon slump at 3 p.m. in the office – only this time you're in bed, it's 2 a.m. and you're stressing that you have to get up in 4 hours.

Try to wean yourself off your pre-bedtime snack habit. If you really need to eat something and/or hunger is disrupting your sleep, a handful of nuts and seeds can be a good choice as they contain L-tryptophan, which promotes the production of serotonin, a neurotransmitter which becomes melatonin as darkness triggers sleep. Tryptophan is found in most protein-based foods – eggs, poultry, meat, fish and cheese. Try a pear dipped in hazelnut butter or a smoothie made from a third of a banana with some coconut milk and a tablespoon of nut butter. Chamomile tea can also have a mild, sedative effect.

Exercise reminder

If your motivation to exercise is flagging by the time you get back from work, fool your brain. Tell yourself you will just do a little 10-minute walk or a 15-minute home circuit class. Once you've started, you will probably do more. If you don't, then you can still celebrate – you have moved your body and that's a habit worth getting into.

Dessert ideas for kids (good for big kids too)

These fun, low-sugar desserts take seconds to make:

Mango and coconut ice lollies

Blend one ripe mango with the juice of one lime and a can of coconut milk. Pour into lollipop moulds and freeze.

Knickerbocker glory

In a tall glass, layer fresh blueberries and raspberries with Greek yoghurt mixed with desiccated coconut. Top with chopped nuts and a drizzle of honey.

Banana sundae

Chop a banana and add scoops of berry ice cream (see recipe later on in this chapter). Top with coconut flakes and a drizzle of good-quality melted chocolate.

Chocolate mousse

Follow the same recipe for adults (see recipe) but blend with the juice of one orange and add slightly more honey for extra sweetness and/or sprinkle with desiccated coconut. For a chocolate mint version, leave out the orange and add some peppermint extract.

Ten tips for a good night's sleep

A good night's sleep lowers levels of ghrelin, the hormone that makes you feel hungry and raises levels of leptin, the hormone that tells your body it's full. The following 12 habits will help you get the best night's sleep and minimise cravings the next day:

1. **Go to bed at the same time each night.** This helps your body get into a sleep rhythm.

2. **Create a relaxing bedtime routine.** Soak in the bath; listen to soothing music; read something spiritual or uplifting; or try relaxation techniques such as breathing, stretching or meditation.

3. **Embrace candlelit dinners.** Too much light prior to bed can suppress the beneficial effects of melatonin. Dim the lights or light some candles. The light from a candle is soft and soothing (there may be a biological reason for that – to our brain, a candle is a mini 'fire').

4. **Stop work.** Stop working at least an hour or two before bed to give your mind time to unwind.

5. **Turn off screens at least an hour before bed.** The blue light emitted from the computers, smartphones and TV screens impedes melatonin production.

6. **Eat a light dinner.** Heavy meals can elevate your metabolic rate and interfere with sleep. Finish eating at least 2–3 hours before hitting the sack.

7. **Avoid stimulants.** Caffeine, cigarettes, sugar and alcohol can all disrupt sleep. Alcohol can initiate sleep but having too many drinks can cause low blood sugar and increased levels of cortisol, resulting in restless or disturbed sleep.

8. **Create a sleep-inducing bedroom.** Ensure your room is dark, quiet, comfortable and cool. While bright lights, heat or noise might not wake you up, they can interfere with the quality of your sleep. Flip your alarm clock round, wear an eye mask, use ear plugs, invest in a blackout shade and/or use a towel to block light coming in under the door.

9. **Exercise regularly.** Exercise improves sleep but avoid exercising late in the evening.

10. **Spend time outdoors during the day.** Light regulates secretion of the sleep-promoting hormone melatonin.

Recipes

The recipes below take seconds to make and require minimal ingredients, but they create desserts that are delicious, creamy and decadent. (It goes without saying that any recipe containing sweeteners, such as honey and dates, should be consumed in moderation.)

Berry ice cream

Serves 2

Ingredients

- 2 handfuls of frozen or fresh berries
- A splash of almond milk
- A spoonful of nut butter

Instructions

Blend all the ingredients, tip into a plastic tub and place in the freezer for 2-4 hours.

Chocolate mousse

Serves 2-3

Ingredients

- 2 very ripe avocados
- 2 tbsp raw cacao powder
- 1 tsp of honey (or sweetener of your choice)

Instructions

Blend all the ingredients and add more cacao powder or honey as needed. Try adding different flavours such as the zest and juice of one orange or a few drops of vanilla extract.

Fried pineapple

Serves 1–2

Ingredients

- 2 slices of pineapple
- Plain or Greek yoghurt

Instructions

Fry the pineapple slices in a little coconut oil and serve with a dollop of yoghurt and a sprinkle of cinnamon.

Coconut pancakes

Makes 6

Ingredients

- 2 eggs
- 2 tbsp coconut oil
- 5 tbsp coconut milk
- ¼ tsp salt
- 2 tbsp coconut flour
- ¼ tsp baking powder
- A handful of your preferred topping, e.g. seeds, blueberries, raspberries

Instructions

Mix everything into a batter using a blender or hand mixer. Let the mixture stand for 5 minutes to thicken. Stir the seeds, blueberries or raspberries into the mixture. Lightly fry a tablespoon of the batter for each pancake. Serve with macadamia cream (see following recipe) and/or berry sauce.

Macadamia cream

Makes 3–4 tablespoons

Ingredients
- Handful of macadamia nuts
- Juice of ½ an orange
- 2 medjool dates
- ¼ vanilla pod

Instructions
Blend everything together and add extra water or coconut milk to gain the desired consistency. The cream will stay fresh in the fridge for about three days.

Berry sauce

Serves 2

Ingredients
- 2 handfuls of mixed berries
- A little grated orange zest, to taste
- A little finely grated ginger, to taste
- A little honey, to taste

Instructions
Place the berries, orange zest and grated fresh ginger in a saucepan and stew, adding a little water if needed. Add a little honey to taste if needed. Serve over ice cream or sorbet.

Final Thoughts

Reducing sugar in your diet is not about being harsh and strict with yourself. Analysing every morsel of food that passes your lips is not a recipe for health and happiness. Equally, nobody wants to be celebrating a birthday or anniversary with a solitary cupcake between family and friends! The occasional sweet treat isn't going to undo all your good work if you're eating a balanced diet. **What matters most is what you do on a day-to-day basis.**

Sugary drinks and processed food are the top sources of added sugar in our diet. This is where to focus your small steps. If swapping your high-sugar breakfast cereal for a low-sugar cereal feels achievable and easy, that's a great place to start. If trying a happy eating technique feels exciting, that's the small step for you. Small steps can seem inconsequential to begin with, but they soon add up:

- Swapping your morning glass of juice for herbal tea saves you 8 teaspoons of sugar.
- Swapping a shop-bought cereal bar for a handful of nuts saves 3 teaspoons.
- Swapping your can of fizzy drink for a glass of sparkling water saves 8 teaspoons.
- Swapping your ready-made meal for a home-cooked version saves 5 teaspoons.

These changes add up to 24 fewer teaspoons of sugar a day. That's 168 teaspoons a week! And that's just four changes; the tip of the iceberg. After three to six months, try retaking the *Are you addicted?* test at the beginning of the book and you'll soon see just how far you have come.

Take a small step. *Celebrate!* Repeat. Get up the next day and do it again.

It's like the old Buddhist saying: 'If you're facing in the right direction, all you have to do is keep walking.'

Resources

If you would like to learn more about the topics covered in this book, the following list contains some inspirational books, websites and DVDs.

Sugar

Gillespie, David *Sweet Poison: Why Sugar Makes Us Fat* (2013, Penguin)

Lustig, Dr Robert *Fat Chance: The Hidden Truth About Sugar, Obesity and Disease* (2014, Fourth Estate)

Perlmutter, David *Grain Brain: The Surprising Truth About Wheat, Carbs, and Sugar – Your Brain's Silent Killers* (2014, Yellow Kite)

Yudkin, John *Pure, White and Deadly* (re-issue 2012, Penguin)

Recipes

Pinnock, Dale *The Medicinal Chef: Eat Your Way to Better Health* and *The Medicinal Chef: Healthy Every Day* (2013, Quadrille)

Wilson, Sarah *I Quit Sugar* and *I Quit Sugar For Life* (2014, Macmillan)

Healthy eating and real food

Pollan, Michael *In Defence of Food: An Eater's Manifesto* (2009, Penguin)

Food Rules: An Eater's Manual (2010, Penguin)

Sisson, Mark *The Primal Blueprint* (2012, Vermilion)

www.marksdailyapple.com

Small steps

Maurer, Robert *One Small Step Can Change Your Life* (2004, Workman Publishing)

Mindfulness

Harrison, Eric *The 5-Minute Meditator: Quick Meditations to Calm Your Body and Mind* (2003, Piatkus)
Puddicombe, Andy *Get Some Headspace: 10 Minutes Can Make All the Difference* (2012, Hodder)
www.getsomeheadspace.com
www.bemindfulonline.com
www.buddhify.com

Yoga DVDs

Ashokananda, Yogi *Power Yoga & Kriya Yoga* (DVD)
Yee, Rodney *AM Yoga for Your Week* (DVD)
Yee, Rodney *Power Yoga Total Body* (DVD)
www.yogaglo.com

Acknowledgements

Thank you to nutritionist and recipe genius Charlotte Hunter, whose down-to-earth, no nonsense approach to food I really respect. She endured several long email and phone conversations, answered my queries about nutrition, and kindly donated the coconut pancakes and macadamia cream recipes for the book. Most importantly, she cast her expert eye over the final manuscript to make sure I wasn't saying anything really stupid. Thank you Charlotte! (**www.charlottehunternutrition.co.uk**)

Thank you also to everyone who took the time to answer my 'sugar survey questions' so frankly and honestly, and who gave their permission to be quoted in the book.

About the Author

Katherine Bassford is a health writer and trainer with a degree in experimental psychology and a masters specialising in human resource management. In 2000, fed up with life as a corporate training consultant, she resigned and qualified as a personal trainer. For the next 12 years she worked as a fitness trainer and set up a business supplying blue-chip companies with articles on employee health and well-being. After obtaining a further diploma in cognitive hypnotherapy, she realised what she *really* wanted to do was move to the coast and write books. She now lives a few minutes' walk from the sea and is working on a follow-up health book and her first children's novel.

www.katherinebassford.com

Bill Statham

WHAT'S *REALLY* IN YOUR BASKET?

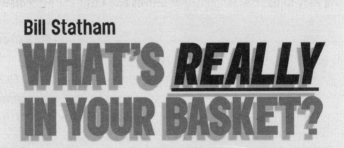

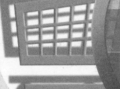

Benzyl salicylate (synthetic)	UV a...
Betaglucans (found in oat fibre and barley)	Thickener
Beta-naphthol (from naphthalene from coal tar)	Solvent

An **easy-to-use** Guide to Food Additives and Cosmetic Ingredients

WHAT'S REALLY IN YOUR BASKET?

An easy-to-use Guide to Food Additives and Cosmetic Ingredients

Bill Statham

£5.99
Paperback
ISBN: 978-1-84024-607-0

Do you REALLY know what's in the products you are buying?

Did you know, for example, that colouring in children's sweets, jelly and soft drinks can potentially cause asthma, skin rash and hyperactivity?

That common ingredients in personal care products like shampoo and toothpaste have been associated with problems ranging from skin irritation to breathing difficulties, nausea, increased risk of cancer and even blindness?

How can you avoid putting harmful additives and chemicals into and onto your body?

This user-friendly guide tells you at a glance which additives are hazardous, which are best avoided and which are safe, making it easier to shop for your family.

Ingredients are listed both alphabetically by chemical and numerically by 'E' number, in colour-coded tables for easy reference.

'Look out for [this book] if you want to know your parabens from your phthalates'
The Times, Body & Soul

50 things you can do today to manage
migraines

Wendy Green

Foreword by Dr Anne MacGregor, Director of Clinical
Research, City of London Migraine Clinic

PERSONAL HEALTH GUIDES

50 THINGS YOU CAN DO TODAY TO MANAGE
MIGRAINES

Wendy Green

£6.99
Paperback
ISBN: 978-1-84024-722-0

*Do you suffer from severe headaches, sometimes with
nausea and visual impairment?*

Can these headaches last for up to a day or longer at a time?

If so, you could be experiencing migraines. In this easy-to-follow book, Wendy
Green explains how dietary, psychological and environmental factors can cause
migraines, and offers practical advice and a holistic approach to help you manage
them, including simple lifestyle and dietary changes and DIY complementary
therapies.

Find out 50 things you can do to today to help you cope with migraines, including:

- Identify your migraine triggers and learn how to manage them
- Discover how to treat children and teenagers with the condition
- Choose beneficial foods and supplements
- Manage stress and relax to reduce attacks
- Learn how to adapt your home and work environments
- Find helpful organisations and products

Have you enjoyed this book?
If so, why not write a review on your favourite website?

If you're interested in finding out more about our books,
find us on Facebook at **Summersdale Publishers** and
follow us on Twitter at **@Summersdale**.

Thanks very much for buying this Summersdale book.

www.summersdale.com